THE
FIT
FOODIE

THE
FIT
FOODIE

Derval O'Rourke

PENGUIN LIFE

AN IMPRINT OF

PENGUIN BOOKS

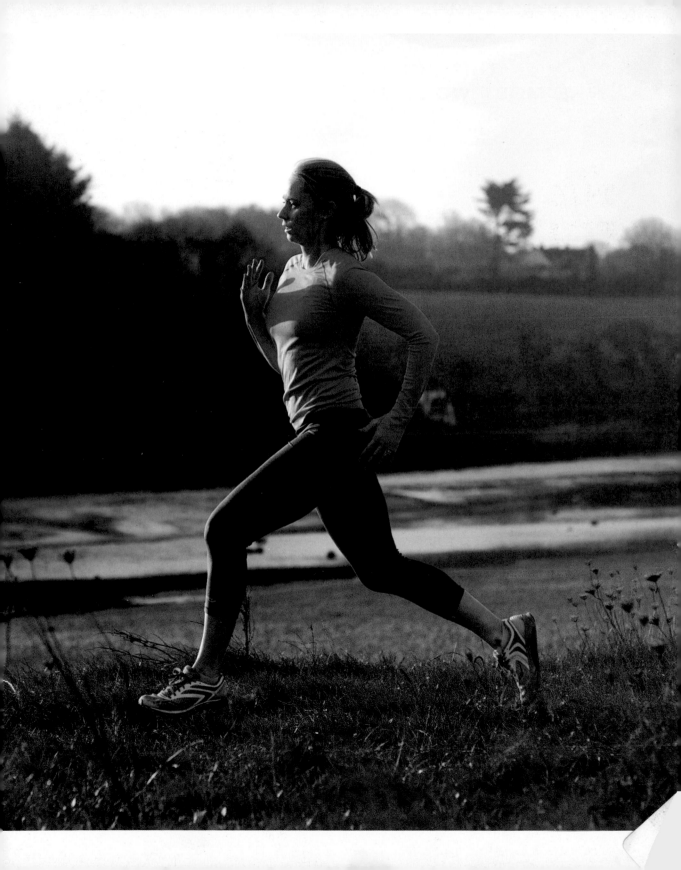

THIS BOOK IS FOR DAFNE.
THE MOST WONDERFUL GIRL IN THE WORLD

PENGUIN LIFE

UK | USA | Canada | Ireland | Australia
India | New Zealand | South Africa

Penguin Life is part of the Penguin Random House group of companies whose addresses
can be found at global.penguinrandomhouse.com.

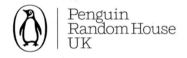

Penguin
Random House
UK

First published 2016
001

Colour reproduction by Rhapsody Ltd
Printed in China

A CIP catalogue record for this book is available from the British Library
ISBN : 978–0–241–97600–5

www.greenpenguin.co.uk

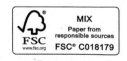

FSC
www.fsc.org

MIX
Paper from
responsible sources
FSC® C018179

Penguin Random House is committed to a sustainable future for
our business, our readers and our planet. This book is made from
Forest Stewardship Council® certified paper.

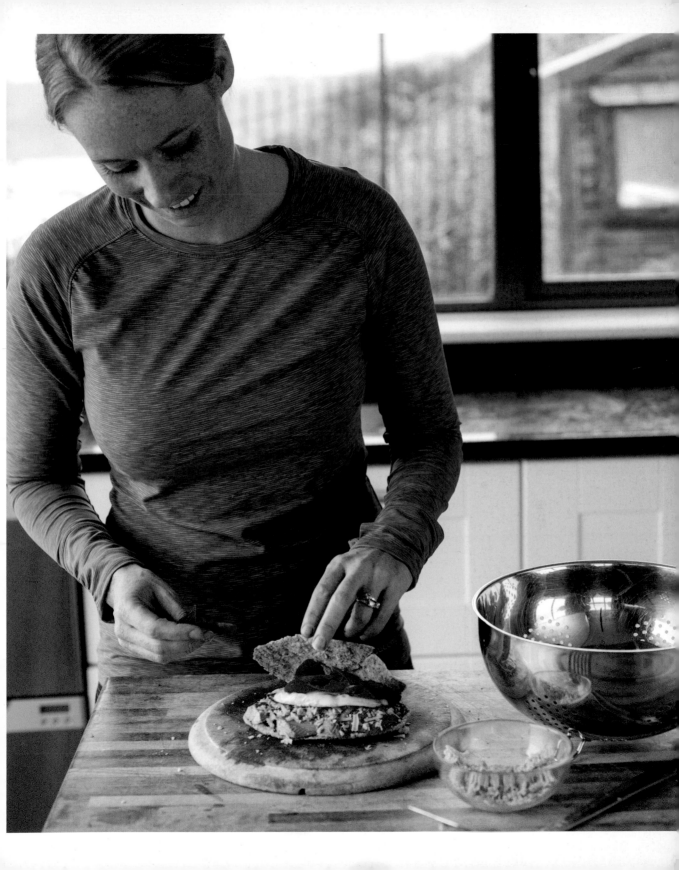

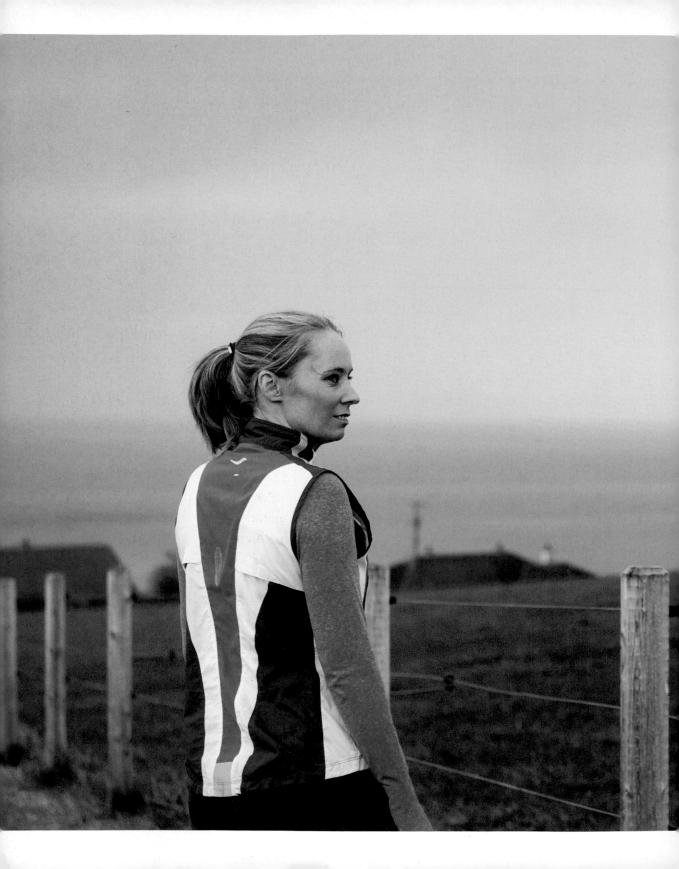

RUNNING ORDER

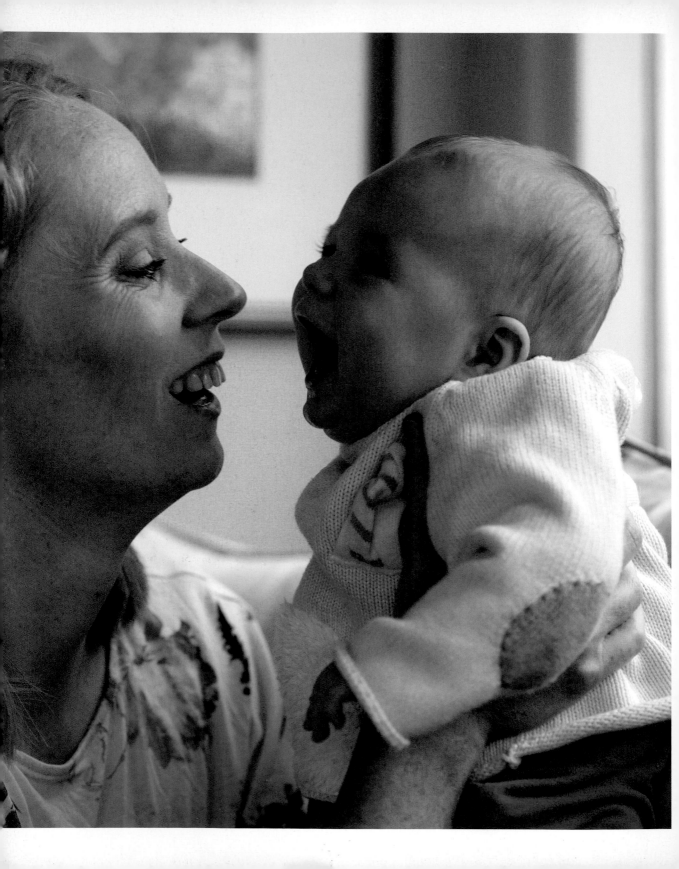

THE JOY OF BEING A FIT FOODIE

Things have changed a lot for me in the past two years. In my old life, I was a professional athlete who travelled the world racing and training. In my new life, I work part-time in professional rugby, part-time running my own company – and on top of all this, I became a mum. In some ways, my old life is unrecognizable.

After retiring I had to take a good look at how I wanted to live. As an elite athlete I had the luxury of being paid to stay fit and healthy and, though I didn't always appreciate it, I was lucky to live that life for twelve years. Being in peak condition was a 24–7 responsibility. There was no clocking off. When I wasn't training or racing, I was thinking about and preparing to train or race. Once I retired, I no longer had to be a specific weight in order to do my job. I no longer needed to stick to a training schedule. There were no big competitions coming up. No more medals to be won. (No TV cameras to face wearing tiny shorts and a crop top!) All of a sudden the obligation to live such a healthy lifestyle was gone.

With the pressure removed I discovered something great: I really loved living a healthy life even when it wasn't my job. While I didn't *have* to be fit, I *wanted* to be fit.

Taking care of my health and fitness became a goal in itself. I wanted to be good to my body: it's the only one I have.

When I lived the elite athlete lifestyle, it wasn't just about work done at the gym or on the track. I took my work into the kitchen. I made sure that I could cook and prepare the foods that would fuel my best performances. Now that I no longer need to think about milliseconds of pace on the track my approach to food can be more relaxed. Nowadays eating is less about performance and more about nourishment and enjoyment. And it's the combination of these two – health and pleasure – that defines Fit Foodie eating and is at the heart of this book. This is a book about eating well and nutritiously. And it's about making good food an easy part of your everyday life so you can be as energized, active and fit as you need and want to be. Whether you are already into fitness, or you simply want to find ways to get into healthier eating and living, I've written *The Fit Foodie* to give you lots of options for all kinds of meals and lots of food for thought on the fitness front too.

In life, there are two things that money can't buy: time and health. I try hard not to be wasteful with either. For me, the best way to do this is to keep things simple in the kitchen. I may not be racing on the track any more, but there are days when I feel like I'm still racing against a clock! I'm sure you do too. Life gets busy. Between family, work and friends, we're all plate-spinning. So my cooking habits have become more practical in recent years and I've learned smart ways to make the best use of my time in the kitchen. For one thing, I make sure to have a well-stocked larder – see 'Fit Foodie Fundamentals' on p. 188. And I'm also a big fan of batch-cooking and freezing – see my freezer tips on p. 128.

Of course it's important to be aware of what you are eating, but it can't take over your life. There are so many opinions out there about the latest 'bad' ingredient that's going to ruin your health or 'good' ingredient that's going to make everything perfect. Being a fit foodie is about cutting through the noise and living according to manageable guidelines. Though I know a good bit about nutrition I'm not an authority, so I asked dietician and performance nutritionist Sharon Madigan to contribute to this book. Sharon works with Olympians, World Champions and high-performance athletes and is a breath of fresh air in terms of sensible and informed advice. See p. 190 for more about Sharon and her explanation of some of the basics of good nutrition. As you'll see, nutrition is not something to fret about. With a little knowledge, you can enjoy your food and nourish yourself at the same time.

Sharon provides a nutritional analysis for every recipe in *The Fit Foodie* – everything except the 'Dessert' section, that is! I think it'd be a shame to nit-pick over the nutritional content of dessert. If you're going to have dessert now and then, go for something delicious and enjoy it. I never feel guilty if I eat cake: I just make sure it's a damn good cake! And if I have a big slice of cake and a cup of coffee with a girlfriend on a Saturday, then I just make sure to get out for some exercise on a Sunday.

A lot of the time, I find myself actually craving foods that are good for me. I look forward to cooking a recipe when I know it's delicious and nutritious. A balanced, practical approach is the only sustainable way to a healthful lifestyle. Strict rules are not for me. Food is there to be enjoyed and it is a wonderful way in which we can nourish ourselves.

One of the greatest compliments I received about my first book, *Food for the Fast Lane*, is that it helped people to learn how to cook. I hope that *The Fit Foodie* will do the same. I'm an enthusiastic home cook who started from a very low knowledge base a little over ten years ago and taught myself from reading and looking at stuff on the internet. When I realized I'd caught the cooking bug, I signed up for a proper intensive cookery course. However you approach it, taking the time to learn some basic cooking skills is invaluable. Take it from me: if you can read, and watch cookery skills demos online, and then just go for it, you can become a decent home cook. I write a little more about this in the 'Doing your homework' section on p. 18.

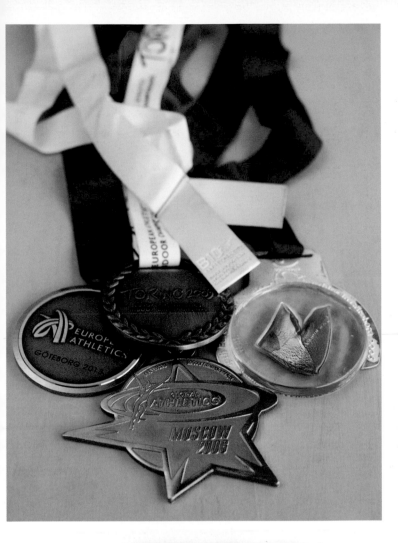
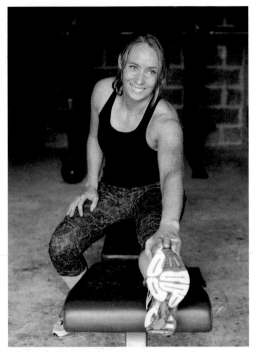
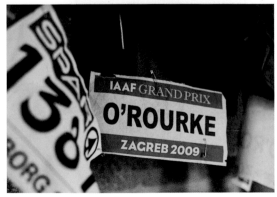
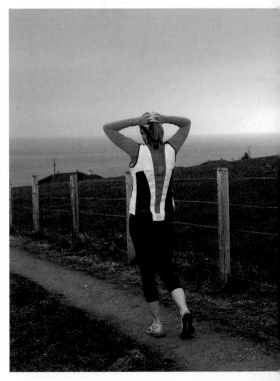

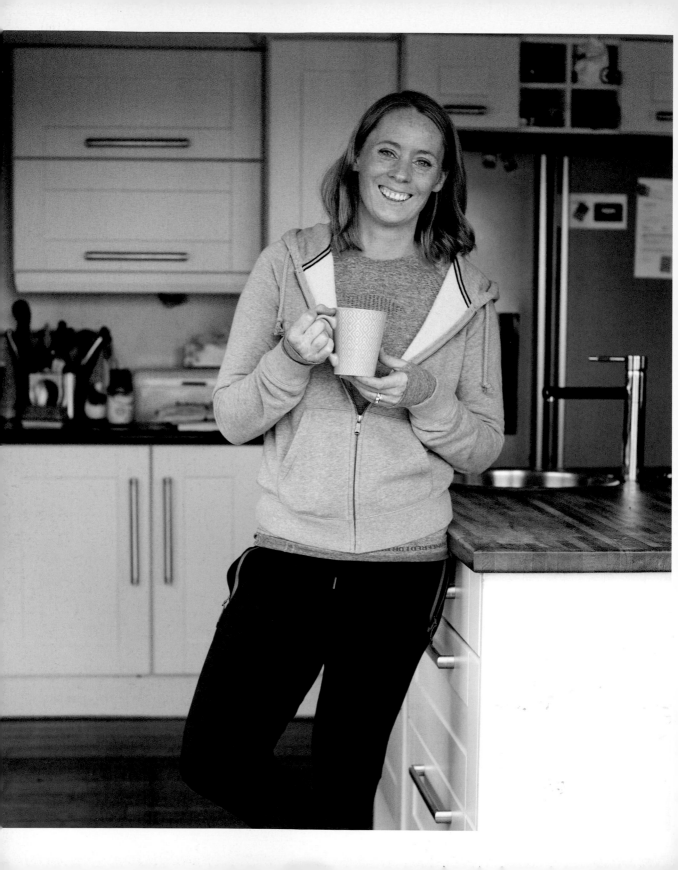

I never regret that decision to lace up the runners and get out for exercise. I find it hugely rewarding every time. Running keeps me healthy and gets me outdoors.

If you are not already into fitness, you might think you're starting from a low base too. But if you can move you can improve your fitness (see some tips in 'Finding new ways to keep fit' on p. 206). I will admit that when it comes to fitness my mindset may be different from other people's. Running has always been a huge part of my identity. When I was a child, I ran all the time. I ran just because I loved the feeling. I loved to put one foot in front of the other and go as fast as I possibly could. And I have never lost that childhood sense of running just for the sheer fun of it. In retirement I realized that I still loved that feeling: it was as much a part of me as being Irish and freckly! So while I stopped training at the same level of intensity according to a structured schedule, I made sure that running was still part of my life.

Apart from running, I also lift weights and stretch. I like it when my body feels strong and flexible. I'm fortunate enough to have weights in my garage and that's where I lift. I don't spend a lot of time weightlifting: 30–40 minutes two or three times a week. Lifting is a great way for me to stay in shape and it's something that I enjoy. I just put on my headphones and get stuck in; it's how I de-stress.

As much as I love running, even I have times when I don't want to go out. Nights after work when it's raining and cold. But I still go out the door. I don't run very far. I go at my own pace and do whatever session I set for myself. I never regret that decision to lace up the runners and get out for exercise. I find it hugely rewarding every time. Running keeps me healthy and gets me outdoors. After a run, my mind is clearer and my mood is brighter. I think I'm a much nicer person to be around afterwards!

I loved my life as a professional athlete and I love my new life. I love learning more about food and fitness. I know the learning will continue for the rest of my life and that excites me. As you read *The Fit Foodie* I hope you can get excited about how simple it is to make changes in your own life. You will see that being a fit foodie is not about setting rigid rules or high-pressure targets. It's not about stressing over fitness and nutrition 24–7. Whether you are trying to win medals, or just be the healthiest, happiest version of yourself you can be, the principles are the same – *Eat Well and Keep Moving*!

RECIPE FOR A FIT FOODIE KITCHEN

As you read through my book, you might wonder how I chose the particular recipes to include. There are **FIVE** things I look at in any recipe before I am happy to award it the Fit Foodie badge.

1 FAST OR FREEZE

You'll see symbols beside many Fit Foodie recipes: FAST and FREEZER.

 THE **FAST** SYMBOL is awarded to recipes that can be made in around 20 minutes: look for this when you want fresh food in a hurry!

 THE **FREEZER** SYMBOL is awarded to recipes that freeze well: look for this when you have the time to batch-cook and stock up your freezer for busy days ahead.

2 INGREDIENTS

Good ingredients form the base of every good meal. I seek out ingredients that are fresh, delicious and nutritious. Fit Foodie recipes are very adaptable, though, so feel free to work with what you've got.

3 GOODNESS IN

I try to include protein (animal or plant-based) with every meal. I keep an eye on saturated fat content. I give a quick hello to calories. Not all calories are created equal – so I don't calorie count but I do watch out for calorie-dense foods. I increase the vitamin and mineral content of meals with fresh fruits and vegetables wherever possible. See p. 190 for more information from Olympic nutritionist Sharon Madigan, who created the Fit Foodie nutrition grids.

4 YOU CAN DO IT!

Cooking from scratch is a big part of Fit Foodie recipes but I promise you: even the most basic skills will get you through. You can do it!

5 TIME

Fit Foodie recipes tell you exactly how long it will take to prepare the ingredients (Prep Time) and to cook (Cook Time). Time is precious: we need to make the most of it.

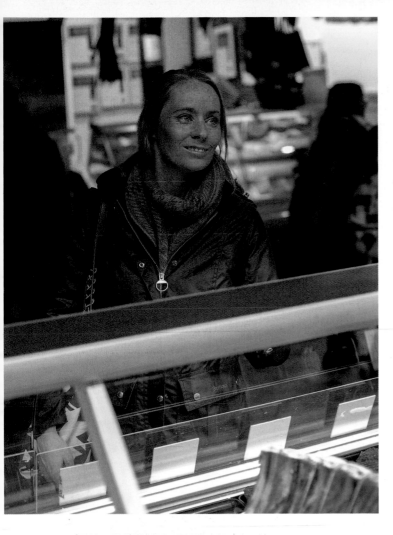
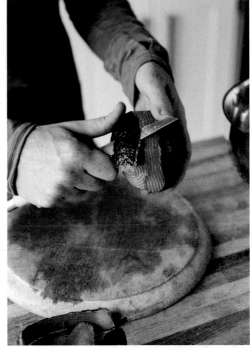
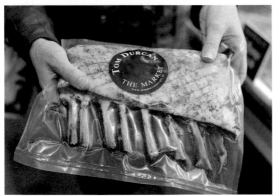
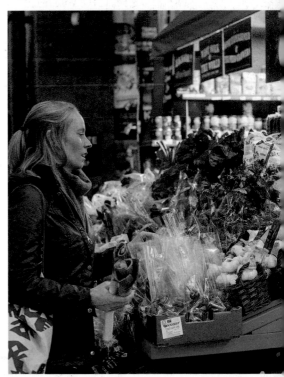

Whether you are trying to win medals, or just be the healthiest, happiest version of yourself you can be, the principles are the same – *Eat Well and Keep Moving!*

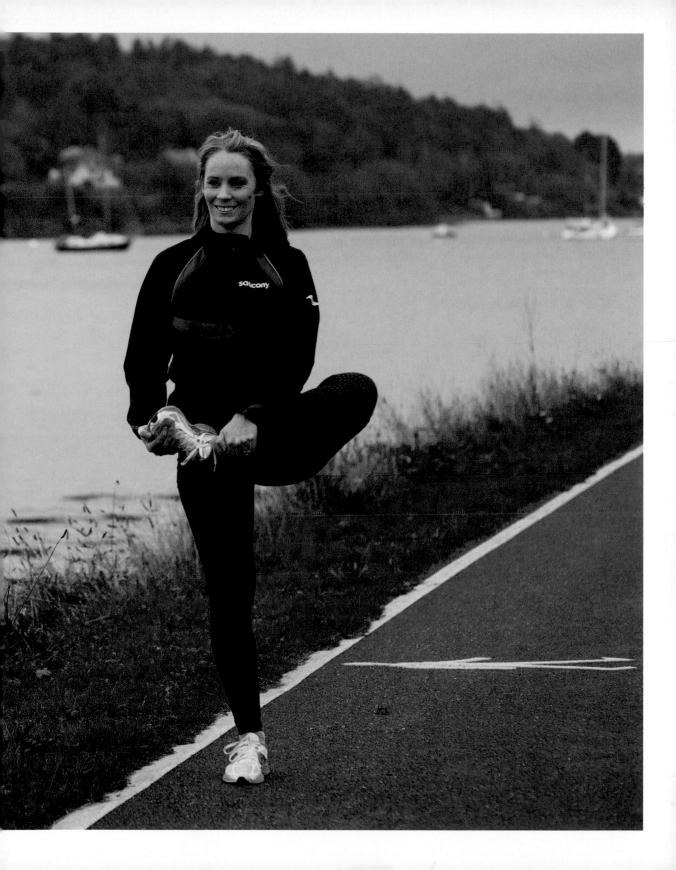

DOING YOUR HOMEWORK

I'm guessing that if you're reading my book, you're not a professional chef. This means that, like me, you sometimes find yourself stumped in the kitchen and in need of help. But that's the fun of cooking: spending time in the kitchen means that we are constantly learning and developing our kitchen skills. It's like doing homework – but fun, interesting homework!

SOLVING PROBLEMS

When you need to solve a problem in the kitchen, the internet is your friend. If you are unsure about an ingredient, do a quick search online: there are probably a million other people who have searched for the exact same thing! I regularly search for alternative ingredients: Can I swap fresh tomatoes for tinned tomatoes? Do I have to use white wine or will something else do? This works in two ways: you will find great ideas for healthy alternatives; and, if a particular ingredient is missing from your larder, you'll still figure out a way to make dinner.

BUILDING SKILLS

Online videos are a great way to build your cooking skills, especially if you're unsure what to do with a specific ingredient. You might not know how to prepare kale or get the seeds out of a pomegranate. You might not know which end is up with an avocado. You might never have heard of a bouquet garni. None of that matters! Just read and watch and learn as you go.

DOING RESEARCH

We are blessed in the internet age. Food websites and blogs can be full of good ideas. When I come across a new recipe online, I tend to look at the reviews from other people who've made the dish. This helps me to quickly decide whether or not it's worth my time to explore further. Some of my favourite websites include www.thekitchn.com and www.bbcgoodfood.com.

LEARNING FROM THE EXPERTS

The people who produce and/or sell food are the experts in how to use it. Make sure that you get out there and talk to the experts. If you're unsure about which cut of meat to use in a particular recipe, chat with your butcher. If you don't know how to prepare fish, ask your fishmonger for help. If you see beautifully fresh vegetables in the greengrocer's or at a farmers' market but you don't know how you'd cook them, talk to the people selling. The answers are out there, so don't be afraid to ask.

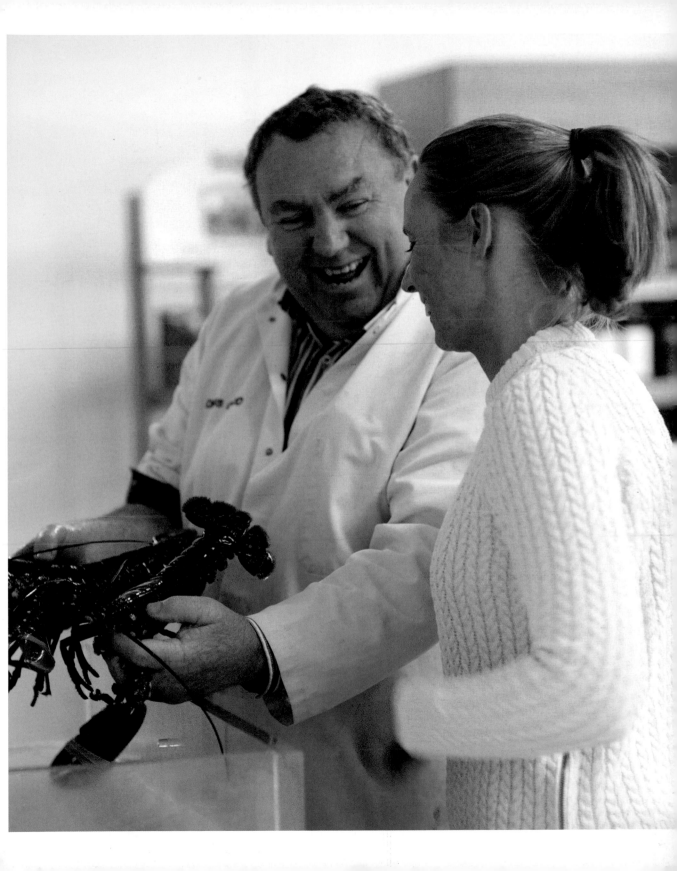

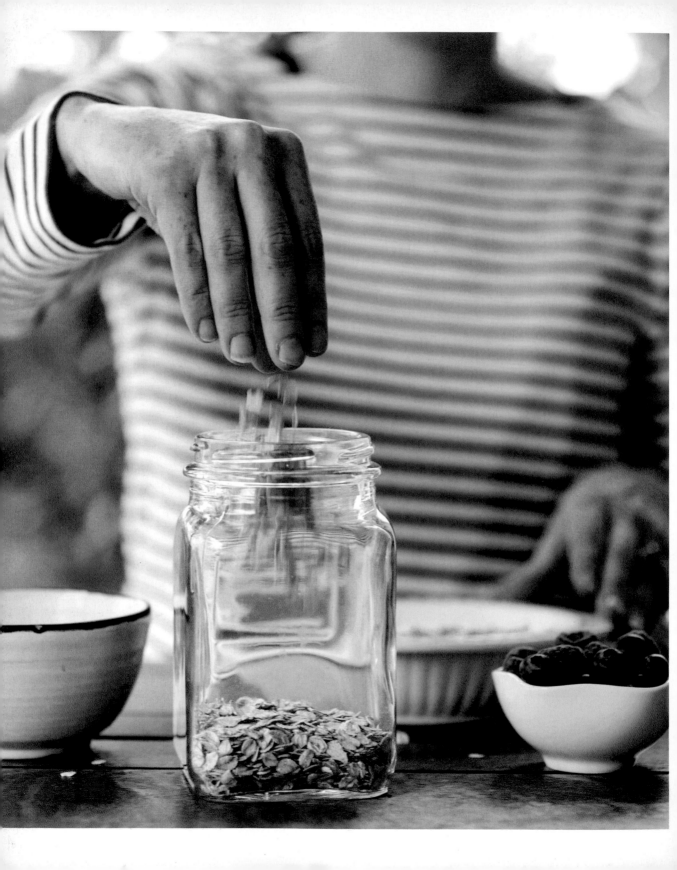

BREAKFAST

OVERNIGHT OATS WITH
RASPBERRY & CHIA

FRUIT-N-NUT GRANOLA

VERY BERRY BREAKFAST SMOOTHIE

FIVE-MINUTE MUESLI

SCRAMBLED EGGS, TWO WAYS

BIG BURRITO BREAKFAST

CHILLI BACON BEANS

THE FITTER PITTA

OVERNIGHT OATS WITH RASPBERRY & CHIA

PREP TIME: 1 MIN (AND OVERNIGHT IN THE FRIDGE)

240ml milk
60g porridge oats
30g frozen raspberries
1 tbsp chia seeds
1 tbsp nuts (pecans work well)
1 tsp agave syrup

Overnight oats are largely responsible for getting me out of bed in the mornings. I love my bed and I need a very good reason to leave it. This breakfast always does the trick! Since these are overnight oats, there's no cooking. You just mix everything together the night before and the recipe takes care of itself. It makes for a great start to the day.

Combine the milk, oats, raspberries and chia seeds in a large bowl. Transfer the mixture to a serving bowl. Cover and leave to soak overnight in the fridge.

Next morning, top with the nuts and agave syrup and serve.

PROTEIN 18.9G

FAT (SATURATED) 28G (8.1G)

CARB 59G

FIBRE 13.5G

CAL 598

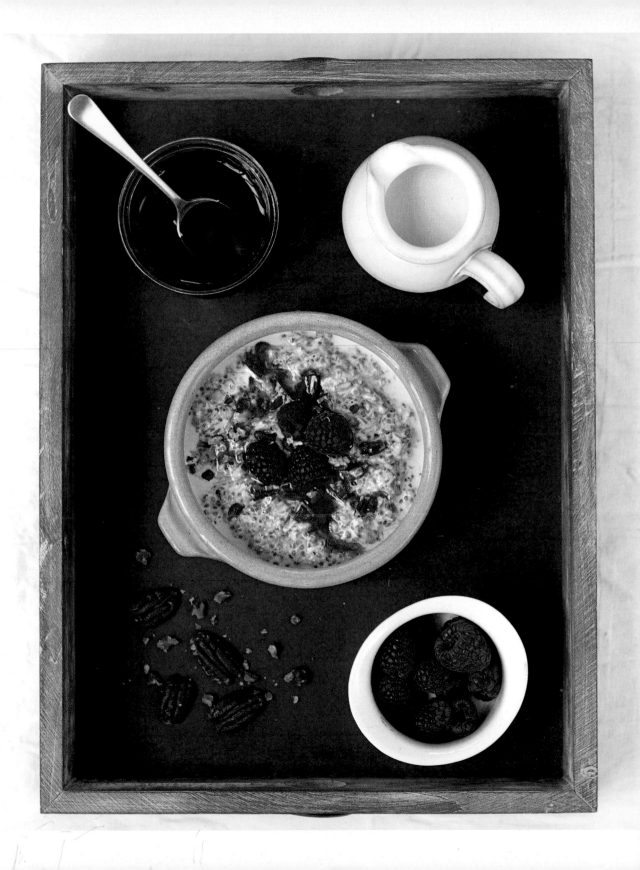

FRUIT-N-NUT GRANOLA

PREP TIME: 5 MIN
COOK TIME: 20 MIN

100g flaked almonds
100g hazelnuts, roughly
  chopped
100g pecans, roughly
  chopped
50g pumpkin seeds
50g sunflower seeds
2 tbsp coconut oil
2 tbsp honey
150g dried fruit (mango
  and apricot work well)

Granola is one of my favourite foods. I try to make one batch a week, normally on a Sunday evening so that I'm ready for the week ahead. Granola is so adaptable: you can eat it for breakfast, as a snack or even as part of a dessert. And it's much better value to make your own granola than to buy it in the shops. If you want to eat this granola before a morning workout, add some extra oats to give you an energy boost!

Preheat the oven to 160°C/325°F/gas 3.

Mix the nuts and seeds in a large bowl. Tip them onto a large baking tray.

Melt the coconut oil in a small pan over a low heat. Stir in the honey. Pour this mixture evenly over the nuts and seeds on the baking tray. Bake for 15 minutes, stirring frequently to ensure that the granola is toasted evenly.

Meanwhile, chop the dried fruit into small pieces. Remove the granola from the oven and stir in the dried fruit pieces. Bake for another 5 minutes, until the dried fruit is nicely chewy.

Remove the granola from the oven and leave to cool. Store the granola in an airtight container, where it will keep for up to two weeks.

PROTEIN 10G	
FAT (SATURATED) 41G (9.6G)	
CARB 23G	
FIBRE 5.2G	
CAL 520	

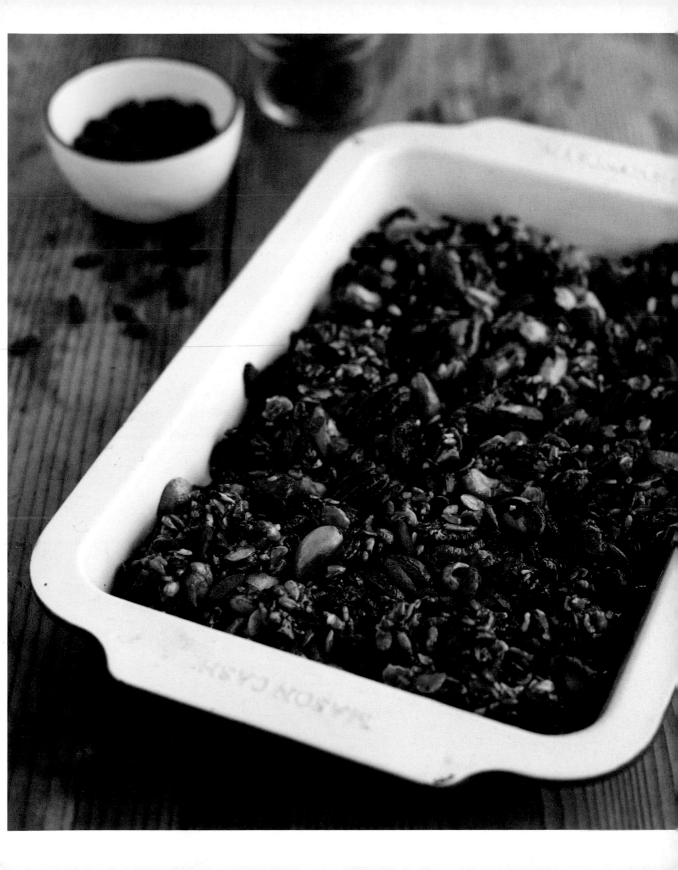

VERY BERRY BREAKFAST SMOOTHIE

300ml apple juice (not from concentrate)
1 ripe banana, peeled
100g mixed (fresh or frozen) berries
1 tbsp chia seeds

This is a great smoothie to have in the morning or after a workout. The chia seeds are full of omega-3, which is good news for your heart. Chia seeds can absorb over ten times their own weight in water, so they work wonders in your digestive system. Just make sure that you drink this smoothie as soon as you make it – before those chia seeds swell up too much! If this smoothie is going to be your full breakfast, throw in a scoop of protein powder to make it more substantial.

Pour the apple juice into a blender and add the banana, berries and chia seeds. Blitz until smooth and creamy. Pour into a tall glass and serve without delay.

PROTEIN 4.2G

FAT (SATURATED) 3.9G (0.4G)

CARB 58G

FIBRE 9.6G

CAL 308

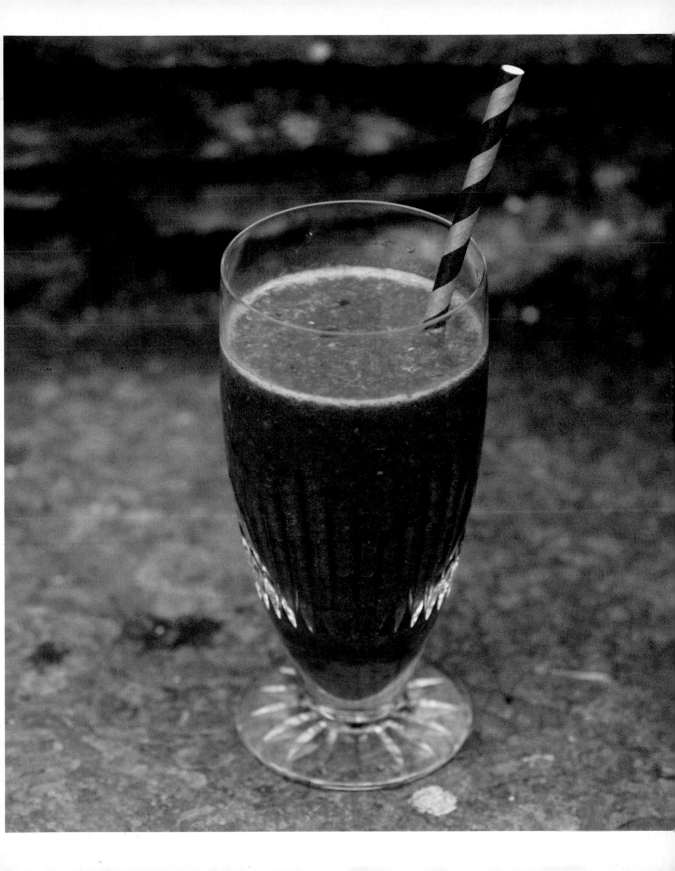

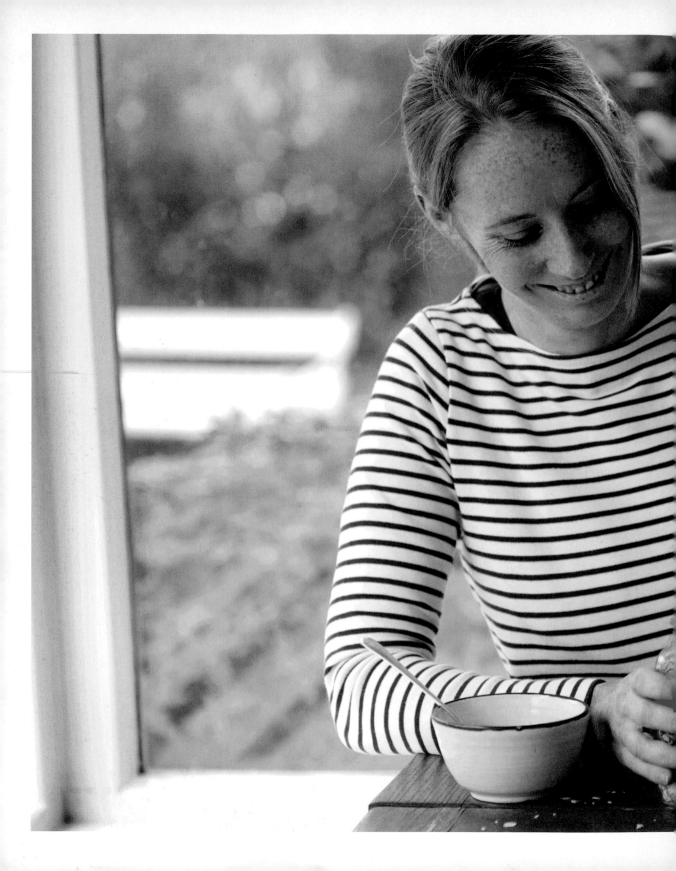

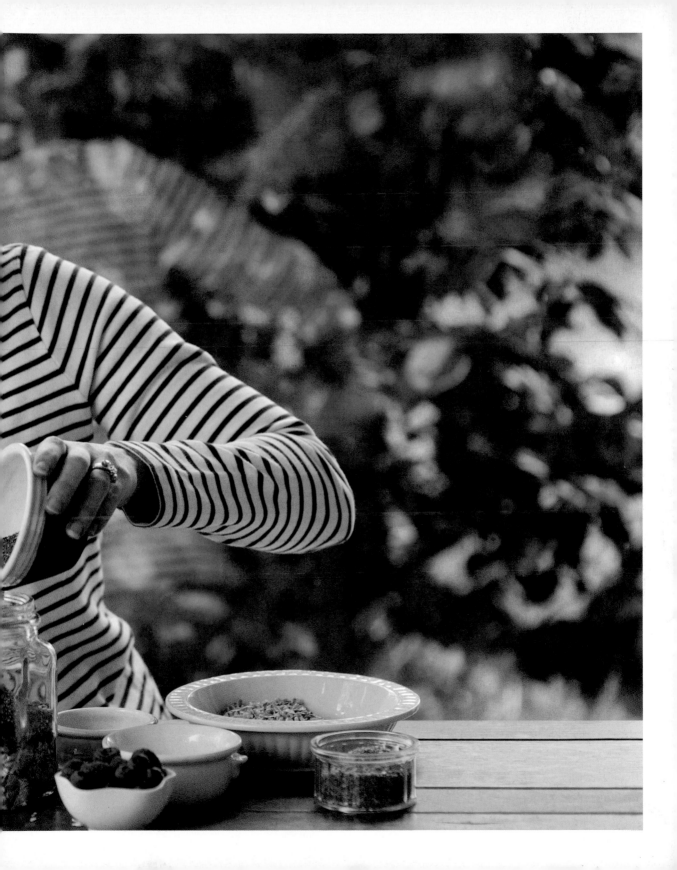

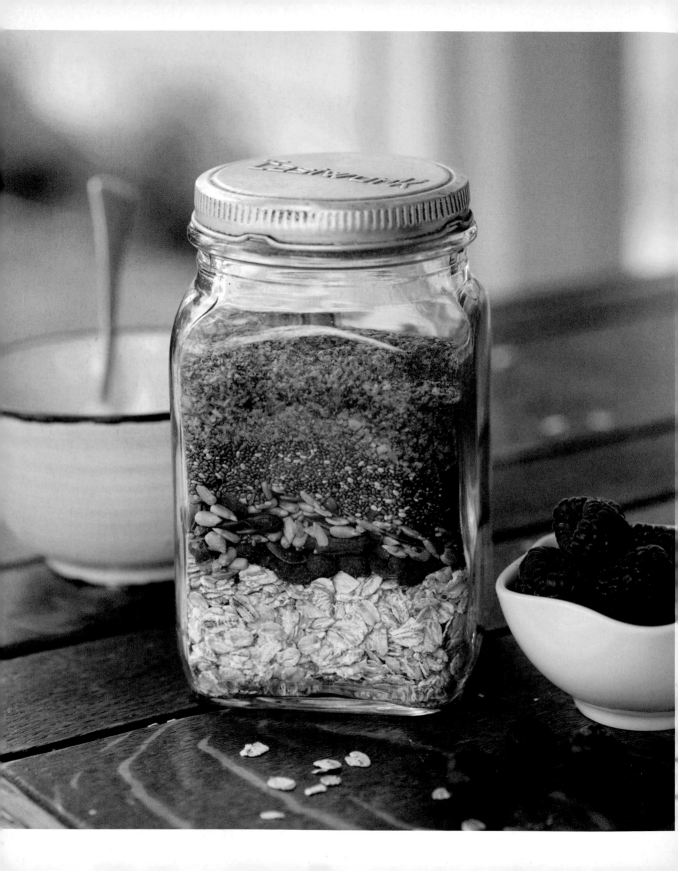

FIVE-MINUTE MUESLI

PREP TIME: 5 MIN

350g jumbo porridge
  oats
150g chia seeds
150g mixed seeds
  (pumpkin and
  sunflower work well)
90g whole dried goji
  berries
90g ground linseed

Shop-bought muesli can be full of sugar and other additives, as well as being overpriced. Take five minutes to make a batch of this muesli instead. It's delicious served with milk or as a topping for fruit and yoghurt. I love to eat it with whatever fresh berries are in season. When it's winter, frozen berries are great – you just need to remember to defrost them the night before! The chia seeds and goji berries are superfoods that will help to support your immune system. And the oats will keep you full all morning. This muesli stores well in an airtight container for about a week.

Mix all of the ingredients in a large bowl. Transfer the muesli to an airtight container.

PROTEIN 19.6G	
FAT (SATURATED) 28G (3.5G)	
CARB 47G	
FIBRE 18.3G	
CAL 557	

SCRAMBLED EGGS, TWO WAYS

I love eggs: they are among the most versatile foods around. There are so many tasty ways to cook eggs for breakfast, lunch or dinner. I particularly like to eat eggs in the morning because the protein sets me up for the day. Scrambled eggs make for a no-fuss cooked breakfast and there are endless ways to vary the flavours and give your breakfast a nutritional boost.

PREP TIME: 2 MIN
COOK TIME: 10 MIN

1 tsp butter
½ small onion, finely chopped
2 eggs, at room temperature
2 tbsp milk
25g white Cheddar, grated
1 tbsp chopped chives
salt and pepper
1 slice of wholemeal toast

THE CHEESE-N-ONION ONE

Melt the butter in a frying pan over a low heat. Add the onion and cook gently for about 5 minutes, until softened. Lightly beat the eggs and milk in a medium bowl. Tip the eggs into the frying pan.

Gently cook the eggs for about 4 minutes, stirring occasionally, until the eggs are thickened and glossy. Spoon the eggs onto a warmed serving plate. Sprinkle over the Cheddar and chives. Season to taste. Serve with a slice of wholemeal toast.

PROTEIN 26G

FAT (SATURATED) 35G (17.2G)

CARB 18.1G

FIBRE 3G

CAL 498

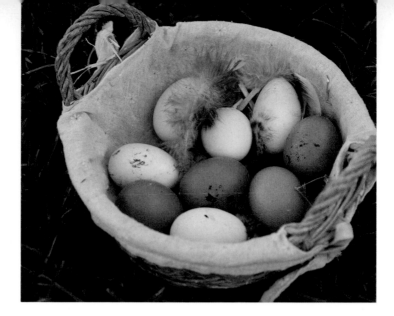

a small handful of kale
   leaves
2 eggs, at room
   temperature
2 tbsp milk
1 tsp butter
25g white Cheddar,
   grated
salt and pepper
1 slice of wholemeal toast

THE KALE ONE

Place 250ml of water in a medium saucepan and bring to the boil. Add the kale and cook, covered, for about 3 minutes, stirring occasionally. Drain and set aside.

Meanwhile, heat a frying pan over a medium heat. Lightly beat the eggs and milk in a medium bowl, add the drained kale and mix well. Tip this mixture into the frying pan.

Gently cook the eggs and kale for 2 minutes, stirring occasionally. Stir in the butter and cook for 2 minutes or until the eggs are thickened and glossy.

Spoon the eggs and kale onto a warmed serving plate. Sprinkle over the Cheddar and season to taste. Serve with a slice of wholemeal toast.

PROTEIN 26G	
FAT (SATURATED) 35G (17G)	
CARB 16.3G	
FIBRE 3.6G	
CAL 492	

BIG BURRITO BREAKFAST

PREP TIME: 5 MIN
COOK TIME: 15 MIN

1 tbsp olive oil
½ onion, finely chopped
2 garlic cloves, crushed
400g tin of mixed beans
1 tbsp butter
5 eggs, beaten
3 tortilla wraps
3 tsp spicy tomato salsa
75g Cheddar, grated

This recipe makes a brilliant late breakfast or brunch after a Sunday morning run. I recommend serving it with a big cup of coffee, a glass of chilled orange juice and a stack of Sunday newspapers. Easy like Sunday morning . . .

Preheat the grill to medium.

Heat the olive oil in a medium pan over a medium heat. Add the onion and garlic and cook for 5 minutes, until softened. Stir in the beans, reduce the heat and leave to simmer while you scramble the eggs.

Melt the butter in a frying pan and pour in the eggs. Cook on a low heat for 3–4 minutes, stirring occasionally, until the eggs are scrambled but still nice and moist. Remove from the heat.

Spoon a third of the bean mixture into the middle of each tortilla wrap. Follow with equal amounts of the scrambled eggs, salsa and Cheddar. Fold the sides of the wraps over the filling, then roll the wraps up from bottom to top to enclose the filling completely. Place the wraps folded-side down on a baking tray. Place under the grill and cook for 2–3 minutes, until lightly toasted, and serve.

PROTEIN 33G
FAT (SATURATED) 33G (12.6G)
CARB 53G
FIBRE 1.9G
CAL 643

SERVES 2

CHILLI BACON BEANS

PREP TIME: 5 MIN
COOK TIME: 10 MIN

1 tbsp olive oil
1 onion, finely chopped
½ red chilli, finely
   chopped
100g bacon, chopped
400g tin of mixed beans,
   drained and rinsed
250ml passata
salt and pepper

These beans can be whipped up in no time at all and they taste fantastic. This is a favourite breakfast of mine after a Saturday morning gym session. Serve the beans with wholemeal toast and a smoothie on the side, and it becomes a feast! The recipe serves two but the beans reheat really well. So if you make this for yourself, you get to enjoy leftovers the next day. And it's not just a breakfast dish, either: I've had many a happy lunchtime with this recipe.

Heat the oil in a large pan over a medium heat. Add the onion and chilli and cook for 2 minutes. Add the bacon and cook for 3 minutes. Stir in the beans and passata and cook for 5 minutes, stirring occasionally, until everything is heated through. Divide the beans between warmed serving plates. Season to taste.

PROTEIN 29G	
FAT (SATURATED) 19.6G (5.2G)	
CARB 44G	
FIBRE 0.9G	
CAL 472	

THE FITTER PITTA

PREP TIME: 5 MIN
COOK TIME: 5 MIN

1 tbsp olive oil
1 egg, at room
  temperature
1 wholemeal pitta
½ avocado, peeled and
  finely sliced
25g white Cheddar,
  grated
a small handful of baby
  spinach

The Fitter Pitta is a toasted pitta packed full of avocado, Cheddar and spinach – all topped off with a fried egg. The avocado gives omega-3 goodness, vitamin K and vitamin C; the egg is full of vitamin B and protein; and the Cheddar gives a nice boost of calcium. It would be hard to find a better start to your day.

Heat the oil in a small frying pan over a low-medium heat. Break the egg into the pan. Gently cook for about 5 minutes, until the white is set but the yolk is still runny.

Meanwhile, toast the pitta on both sides. Split open and stuff with the avocado, Cheddar and spinach. Top with the fried egg and serve.

PROTEIN 22G

FAT (SATURATED) 43G (12.5G)

CARB 37G

FIBRE 8.8G

CAL 645

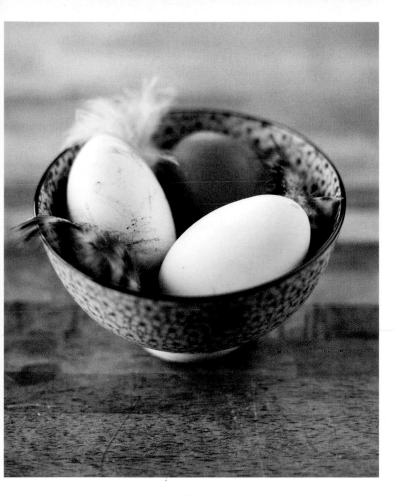

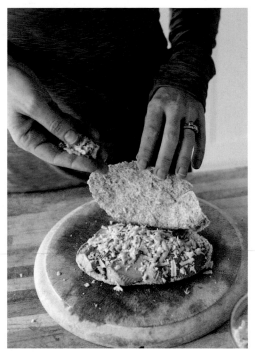

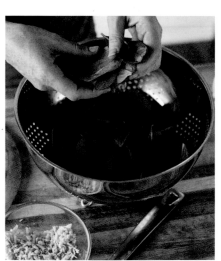

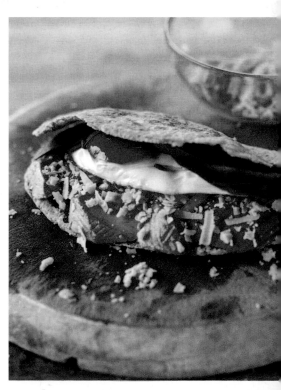

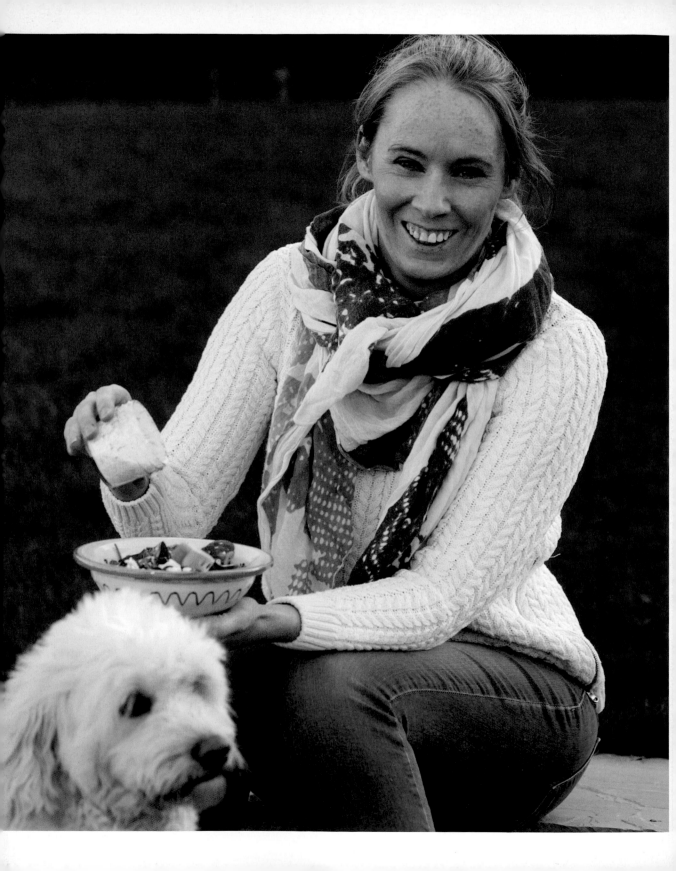

LUNCH

FIT FOODIE NOODLE POTS

NO-DOUGH PIZZAS

CHICKEN & CHUTNEY POCKETS

HOT CHICKEN SANDWICH

SPINACH & FETA FRITTATA

TWO-FISH MISHMASH

QUICK BAKED POTATO & TUNA

GET-YOUR-GREENS SOUP

LEEK & POTATO SOUP

TOMATO & RED LENTIL SOUP

PEA & MINT SOUP

SUMMER COUSCOUS SALAD

TUNA & QUINOA SALAD

ROCKET, FENNEL & ORANGE SALAD

CRUNCHY BROCCOLI & FETA SALAD

QUINOA SALAD WITH TOASTED

NUTS & BLUE CHEESE

THREE-GRAIN SALAD

THREE-BEAN SALAD

TUNA PESTO PASTA

FIT FOODIE NOODLE POTS

PREP TIME: 10 MIN
COOK TIME: 3 MIN

THE MILD ONE

150g straight-to-wok rice noodles
2 small florets of broccoli
1 scallion, finely sliced
¼ carrot, peeled and grated
A few peas (preferably fresh but frozen will work)
a thumb-sized piece of fresh ginger, grated
a few spinach leaves
1 tsp vegetable stock powder

THE SPICY ONE

150g straight-to-wok rice noodles
a handful of shredded cooked chicken
5 sugar snap peas, halved
1 scallion, finely sliced
a few beansprouts
½ tsp chopped chilli
1 tbsp soy sauce
1 tsp vegetable stock powder

Fit Foodie Noodle Pots are a lot of fun! They make for healthy, portable hot lunches. All you have to do is gather your ingredients in a preserving jar (such as Kilner or Le Parfait) and then store it in the fridge. When lunchtime comes around, you just boil the kettle and pour the hot water into the jar. Before you know it, your Fit Foodie Noodle Pot is ready to go.

You will need a large sterilized preserving jar that allows you room to stir. Place all of the ingredients in the jar and store in the fridge until needed. Just before serving, pour 200ml of boiling water into the jar. Stir well to combine the ingredients and soften the noodles. Enjoy!

THE MILD ONE	
PROTEIN 13.2G	
FAT (SATURATED) 1.7G (0.4G)	
CARB 121G	
FIBRE 7.5G	
CAL 570	

THE SPICY ONE	
PROTEIN 61G	
FAT (SATURATED) 4.2G (1.1G)	
CARB 118G	
FIBRE 2.7G	
CAL 761	

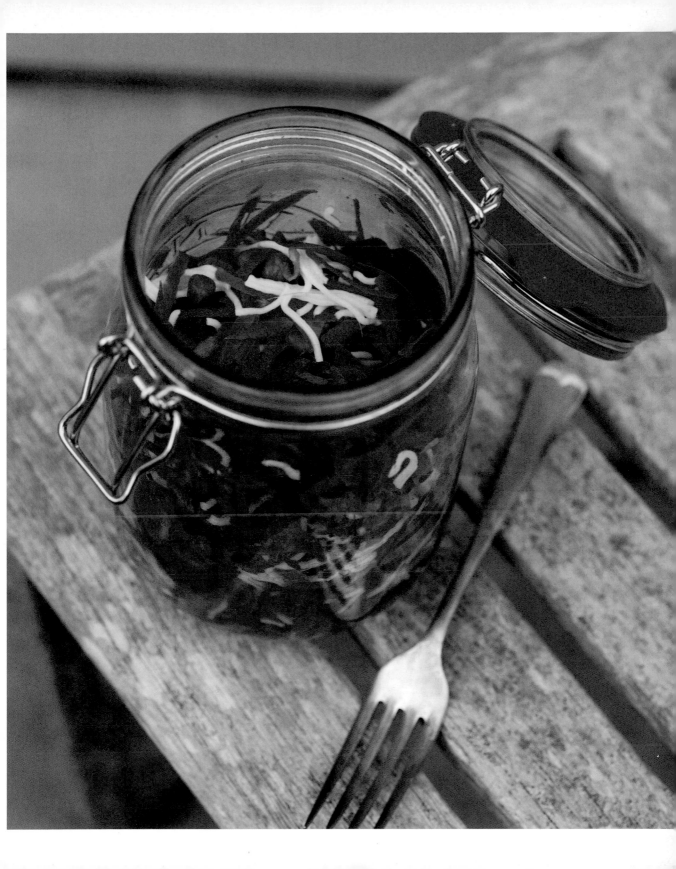

NO-DOUGH PIZZAS

No-Dough Pizzas are great when you want a savoury pizza flavour but you don't want to eat stodge. Tortilla wraps make an ideal base for quick lunchtime pizzas. No-Dough Pizzas are ready in minutes and are a big hit with everyone. In the little time it takes for the pizzas to cook, you could make a nice green salad to serve on the side.

THE MEAT ONE

PREP TIME: 20 MIN
COOK TIME: 7-10 MIN

1 tortilla wrap
1 tsp olive oil
1 tsp finely chopped onion
150g minced lamb
1 tbsp basil pesto
1 jalapeño pepper, finely chopped
1 tbsp natural yoghurt
a small handful of mint leaves, chopped
a small handful of rocket

Preheat the oven to 180°C/350°F/gas 4. Line a baking sheet with parchment paper. Place the tortilla wrap on the baking sheet.

Heat the oil in a medium pan over a medium heat. Add the onion and cook for 2 minutes. Add the mince and cook for 15 minutes or until cooked through.

Use the back of a spoon to spread the pesto over the tortilla wrap. Spread the cooked mince on the pizza. Scatter over the jalapeño pepper and dot the pizza with natural yoghurt. Bake for up to 10 minutes.

Cut the cooked pizza into slices and place on a warmed serving plate. Scatter over the mint. Top with the rocket and serve.

PROTEIN 45G	
FAT (SATURATED) 40G (12.7G)	
CARB 33G	
FIBRE 3.4G	
CAL 680	

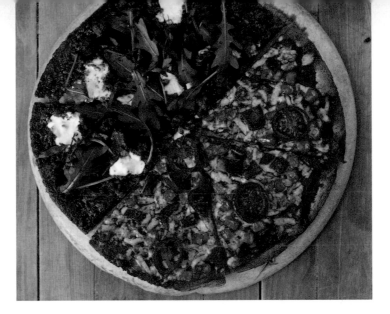

THE VEGETARIAN ONE

PREP TIME: 3 MIN
COOK TIME: 7-10 MIN

1 tortilla wrap
2 tbsp passata or tomato
  purée
2 drops of Tabasco sauce
3 cherry tomatoes,
  halved
½ red pepper, chopped
1 tbsp sweetcorn
25g Cheddar, grated

Preheat the oven to 180°C/350°F/gas 4. Line a baking sheet with parchment paper. Place the tortilla wrap on the baking sheet.

Mix the passata and Tabasco in a small bowl. Use the back of a spoon to spread this mixture over the tortilla wrap. Scatter over the tomatoes, pepper and sweetcorn. Sprinkle over the Cheddar. Place the pizza in the oven and bake for up to 10 minutes, until the cheese is golden and bubbling. Cut the cooked pizza into slices and place on a warmed serving plate.

PROTEIN 16.6G

FAT (SATURATED) 14.4G (6.7G)

CARB 41G

FIBRE 3.1G

CAL 369

CHICKEN & CHUTNEY POCKETS

PREP TIME: 3 MIN
COOK TIME: 7 MIN

FOR THE DRESSING
2 tbsp natural yoghurt
1 tsp Ballymaloe relish
  (or another fruity
  chutney)
2 scallions, finely sliced
1 tbsp chopped chives
salt and pepper
1 tbsp olive oil
1 skinless chicken breast
  fillet, cubed
2 pittas
25g Cheddar, grated

These pitta pockets are fruity, savoury and can really liven up a lunchtime. They're ready in minutes and taste equally delicious hot or cold. For a hot lunch at home, follow the recipe below. But if you want to prep this for lunch at work, cook the chicken, assemble the dressing and grate the cheese the night before. Store them separately in the fridge until needed. The next day, you just need to find a toaster for the pitta and lunch takes care of itself!

Mix all of the ingredients for the dressing in a small bowl. Season and set aside.

Heat the oil in a medium pan over a medium heat. Cook the chicken for 5 minutes or until cooked through. Drain the chicken. Toast the pittas on both sides. Split open and stuff with the chicken and dressing. Top with the Cheddar and serve.

PROTEIN 38G	
FAT (SATURATED) 14.5G (5.2G)	
CARB 47G	
FIBRE 4.7G	
CAL 481	

HOT CHICKEN SANDWICH

PREP TIME: 30 MIN
COOK TIME: 20 MIN
MAKES: 4 CHICKEN BREASTS

4 skinless chicken breast fillets
2 tbsp maple syrup (or honey)
2 tbsp Worcester sauce
1 tbsp Dijon mustard
2 tsp smoked paprika

PREP TIME: 5 MIN

2 slices of good brown bread
1 breast of Marinated Chicken, still warm from the oven, sliced
½ red pepper, finely sliced
a handful of rocket leaves
a few thin slices of cucumber
1 tbsp natural yoghurt

Chicken sandwiches can sometimes be dull, but I promise you that this one is not! It's actually good enough to eat as a light supper when you need something warm, satisfying and easy after a hard day. The marinated chicken is great for stocking up your fridge. It takes less than an hour to make and it gives you endless options for the days ahead. I'll usually have a batch of this marinated chicken on the go so that I'm not stuck for a sandwich-filler, salad-topper or post-workout protein snack.

MARINATED CHICKEN

Place all of the ingredients in a large ziplock bag. Press the air out of the bag and seal it securely. Lay the bag on a large plate and use your hands to massage the marinade into the chicken. Leave to marinate at room temperature for 30 minutes. Preheat the oven to 180°C/350°F/gas 4. Remove the chicken breasts from the bag and place them in an ovenproof dish. Roast for 20 minutes or until the chicken is cooked through. Store the cooked chicken in an airtight container in the fridge, where it will keep for several days.

CREATING THE HOT CHICKEN SANDWICH

Place the brown bread slices on a serving plate, side by side. Arrange the chicken slices on top of the bread. Top with the pepper, rocket and cucumber. Finish with a dollop of natural yoghurt and serve.

PROTEIN 61G
FAT (SATURATED) 7.2G (2.1G)
CARB 38G
FIBRE 6.2G
CAL 478

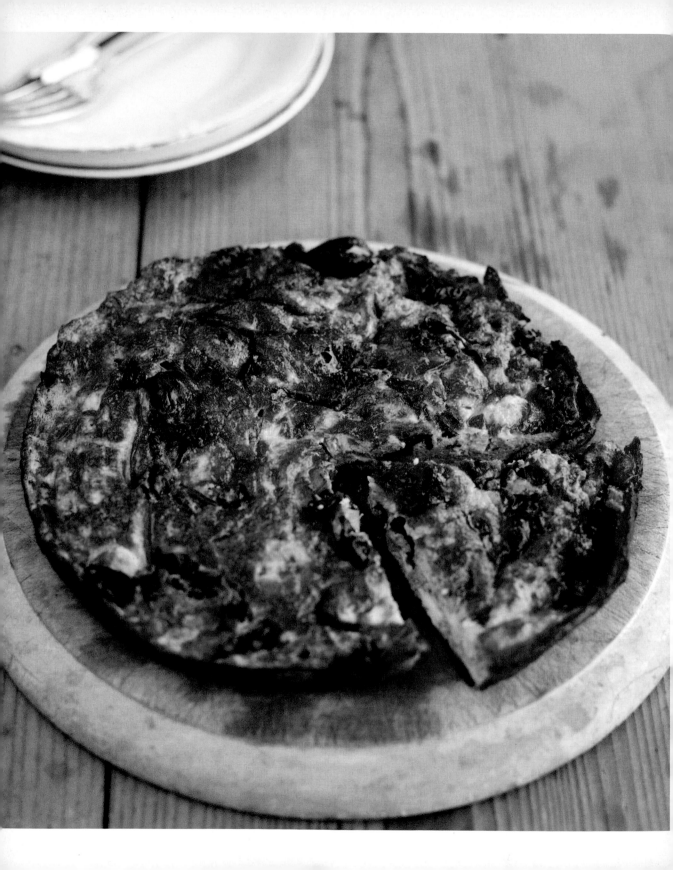

SERVES 2

SPINACH & FETA FRITTATA

PREP TIME: 5 MIN
COOK TIME: 15 MIN

6 eggs
50g feta, diced
4 tbsp milk
a handful of basil leaves,
   torn
salt and pepper
1 tbsp butter
½ onion, finely chopped
a handful of baby
   spinach leaves

This frittata tastes delicious at any time of day. It's perfect for lunch – but if you want to serve it with toasted pitta and a side salad, it becomes a lovely light dinner. I sometimes have it as a leisurely weekend breakfast too. You don't need to fuss too much about the ingredients. If you don't have baby spinach leaves, frozen spinach works well. Frittatas really are endlessly adaptable.

Preheat the grill to a high heat.

Lightly beat the eggs, feta, milk and basil in a medium bowl. Season well.

Heat the butter in a large ovenproof frying pan over a medium-high heat. Cook the onion and spinach for about 5 minutes.

Reduce to a low heat and pour the eggs into the pan. Do not stir the eggs: just allow them to cook gently for about 10 minutes.

When the frittata is softly set and golden underneath, remove the pan from the heat. Place the pan under the grill for a few minutes and cook until the top of the frittata is set and golden.

Cut the frittata into slices and serve on warmed plates.

PROTEIN 27G	
FAT (SATURATED) 31G (13G)	
CARB 4.5G	
FIBRE 0.9G	
CAL 408	

TWO-FISH MISHMASH

PREP TIME: 5 MIN
COOK TIME: 30 MIN
(INCLUDES COOLING)

2 × 100g salmon fillets,
   skinned
180g cod fillet, skinned
3 tbsp natural yoghurt
2 tbsp chopped fresh dill
   (or 1 tsp dried dill)
juice of 1 lime
a few drops of Tabasco
   sauce (optional)
1 ripe avocado, peeled
   and finely chopped

Two-Fish Mishmash makes a delicious light lunch – but you could also eat it for dinner if you serve it with rice and a green salad. I usually double this recipe, so that I can stock up on the Fish Mishmash. It keeps for several days in an airtight container in the fridge and it's also delicious in sandwiches, on baked potatoes or with a simple slice of toast.

Preheat the oven to 180°C/350°F/gas 4. Place the fish fillets in a large ovenproof dish and fill the dish with water. Cover the dish with foil and bake the fish for 20 minutes or until cooked through. Remove the cooked fish to a plate and set aside to cool for 10 minutes.

Use a fork to gently flake the cooked fish into a large bowl. Add the yoghurt, dill, lime juice and Tabasco and mash well.

Arrange the chopped avocado in a neat layer on each serving plate. Top with the Fish Mishmash and serve.

PROTEIN 47G	
FAT (SATURATED) 33G (7.2G)	
CARB 6.3G	
FIBRE 4.2G	
CAL 522	

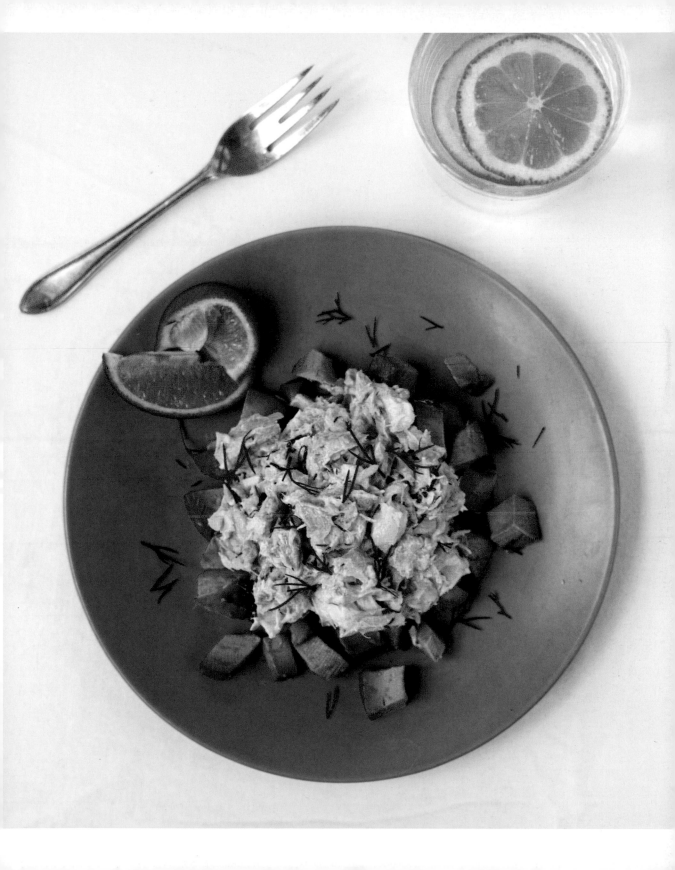

QUICK BAKED POTATO & TUNA

COOK TIME: 10 MIN

1 baking potato
olive oil
salt and pepper
112g tin of tuna in olive
   oil, drained
1 scallion, finely sliced
1 tbsp natural yoghurt
25g Cheddar, grated

This is a lunch I turn to when I know I'll have a busy afternoon that's likely to include a workout. I need something substantial enough to get me through but I can't take hours to make it. So I call on the microwave for a baked potato. The potato gives me carbohydrates for energy and the tuna gives me protein for muscle recovery. It's a winning combo when you're in a hurry. Of course, you can still make this recipe if you don't have a microwave. The oven-baked potato will take longer, but the final result will be equally delicious!

Rub the potato with a little olive oil and sprinkle over some salt. Prick the potato all over with a fork. Place the potato in a microwave-proof dish. Cook at full power for 5 minutes. Turn over the potato and cook for 3–5 minutes more, until soft.

Meanwhile, mix the tuna, scallion and yoghurt in a large bowl. Season to taste and set aside.

Split the baked potato in half lengthways and fill with the tuna mixture. Sprinkle over the Cheddar and serve.

PROTEIN 49G	
FAT (SATURATED) 22G (7.6G)	
CARB 91G	
FIBRE 9.4G	
CAL 776	

GET-YOUR-GREENS SOUP

PREP TIME: 10 MIN
COOK TIME: 20 MIN

2 tbsp butter
1 onion, finely chopped
3 leeks, finely sliced
300g broccoli, broken into florets
200g kale, tough stalks removed
500ml vegetable stock
salt and pepper

Soup is a smart way to up your veggie intake without having to overthink things. I cook soup in big batches and freeze it in individual portions so that I'm never stuck for a nutritious lunch or light dinner. This soup helps to combat inflammation, so it's a great one to eat if you're training hard. Make this soup and you will definitely get your greens!

Melt the butter in a large pan over a low heat. Add the onion and leeks and cook for 5 minutes, until softened. Add the broccoli and kale, stir well and cover. Cook for 5 minutes, stirring occasionally. Add the stock and bring to the boil. Reduce the heat and simmer, covered, for 10 minutes or until the vegetables are tender.

Take the pan off the heat. Purée the soup with a hand blender until smooth. Season to taste and ladle the soup into warmed serving bowls.

PROTEIN 13.2G
FAT (SATURATED) 3.9G (0.7G)
CARB 14.8G
FIBRE 13.3G
CAL 179

LEEK & POTATO SOUP

PREP TIME: 10 MIN
COOK TIME: 25 MIN

3 tbsp coconut oil
4 celery sticks, finely
  chopped
4 garlic cloves, crushed
1 onion, finely chopped
2 leeks, trimmed and
  finely sliced
1 tsp fresh thyme leaves
3 potatoes, peeled and
  diced
600ml vegetable stock
300ml milk
salt and pepper
2 tbsp chopped chives

I'm not sure there is anything more comforting on a cold winter's night than a bowl of this soup. It tastes especially good if you've just come home from a workout and you need a warm and nourishing pick-me-up. Since it's more substantial than most soups, you could use it as a basis for dinner. If I've been out for a run in the rain, this is the soup I'll crave. It's delicious with brown bread and roast chicken on the side. And it's a soup that freezes and reheats beautifully.

Melt the coconut oil in a large pan over a medium heat. Add the celery, garlic and onion and cook for 5 minutes, until softened. Add the leek and thyme and cook for 4 minutes, stirring frequently. Add the potatoes and stock and stir well. Cover and simmer for 15 minutes, until the potatoes are tender.

Remove from the heat and stir in the milk. Purée with a hand blender until smooth. Season to taste and ensure that the soup is heated through. Ladle the soup into warmed serving bowls and sprinkle over the chives.

PROTEIN 6.6G

FAT (SATURATED) 5.4G (3.6G)

CARB 23G

FIBRE 5.6G

CAL 182

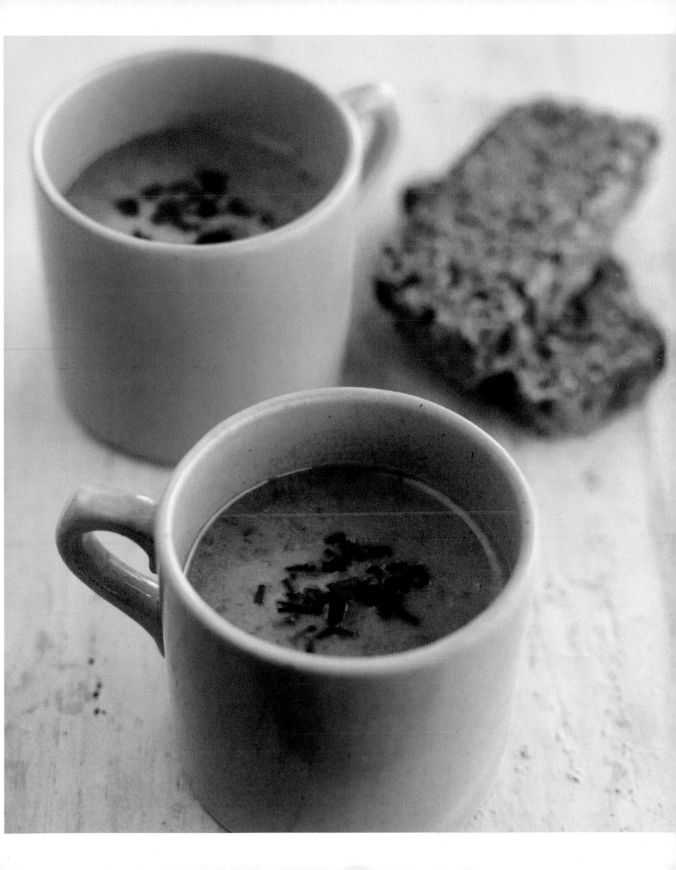

SERVES 4

TOMATO & RED LENTIL SOUP

PREP TIME: 5 MIN
COOK TIME: 35 MIN

1 tsp olive oil
1 onion, finely chopped
4 celery sticks, sliced into
   1 cm pieces
3 carrots, peeled and
   sliced into 1 cm rounds
1 litre vegetable stock
100g dried split red
   lentils
2 bay leaves (or a
   bouquet garni)
500ml passata
salt and pepper

Even when I feel as if there is nothing in the cupboards,
I usually have what's needed to make this soup. It needs no
fancy vegetables, which is proof that a good soup can be
as straightforward as it is delicious. This soup is a real
winter warmer and it's incredibly filling. It packs nutritional
punch with plenty of carotenoids (which come from the
deeply coloured carrots and the tomatoes in the passata).
And you don't even need a blender to make this soup;
it really could not be easier.

Heat the olive oil in a large pan over a low heat. Add the onion, cover, and cook
for about 3 minutes, stirring occasionally. Stir in the celery and carrots and
cook, covered, for another 5 minutes. Add a splash of water if the pan gets dry.

Add the stock, lentils and bay leaves. Stir well and increase the heat to medium.
Simmer, uncovered, for 20 minutes.

Remove the bay leaves and stir in the passata. Simmer for about 10 minutes,
until the vegetables are tender and the passata is heated through. Season to
taste. Ladle the soup into warmed serving bowls.

PROTEIN 10.2G
FAT (SATURATED) 4.4G (0.6G)
CARB 30G
FIBRE 4.3G
CAL 211

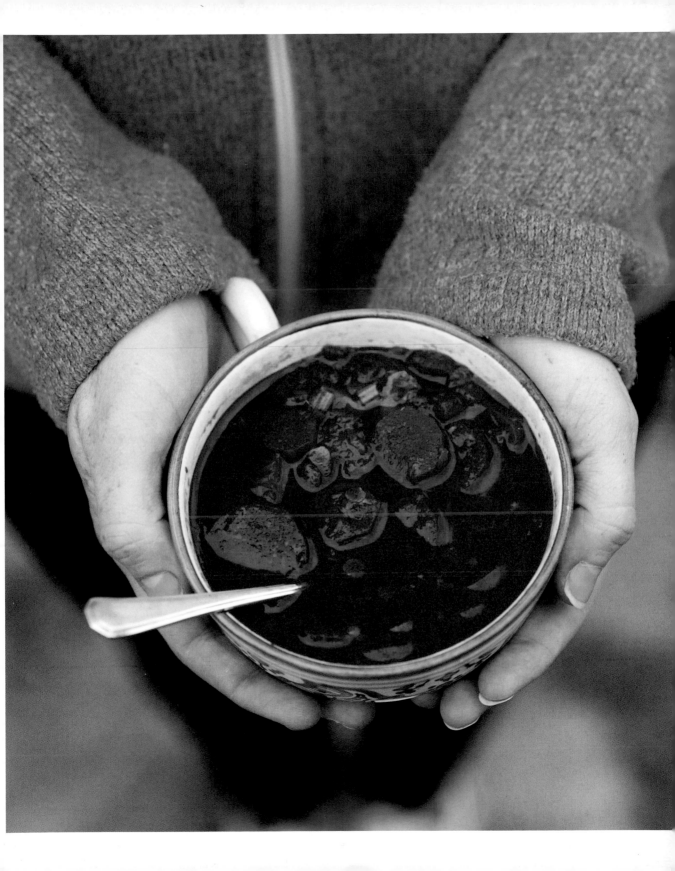

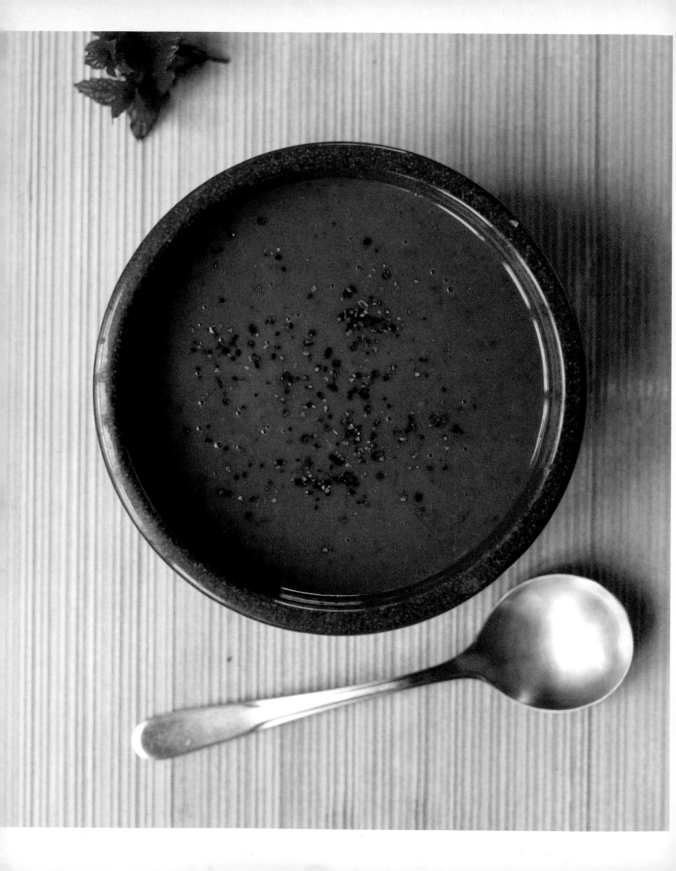

SERVES 5

PEA & MINT SOUP

PREP TIME: 5 MIN
COOK TIME: 15 MIN

1 tbsp butter
1 onion, finely chopped
a handful of mint leaves,
  chopped
800g baby peas
  (preferably fresh, but
  frozen will work)
700ml vegetable stock,
  simmering
freshly ground pepper

It took me a while to get used to the idea of eating green soups: to me they always looked a bit too . . . well . . . green. But then I discovered that pea soup is actually delicious. This soup is a real 'souper hero'! The ingredients are inexpensive, it's tasty, packed full of nutrition and great to cook in a big batch for freezing and reheating. This is delicious by itself and it also goes well with crusty wholemeal bread.

Heat the butter in a large pan over a low heat. Add the onion and mint and cook for about 5 minutes. Stir in the peas and stock and bring to a boil. Simmer, uncovered, for 10 minutes or until the peas are cooked through. Remove from the heat and set aside to cool for a few minutes.

Use a hand blender to blitz the soup. Ladle the soup into warmed serving bowls.

PROTEIN 10.7G	
FAT (SATURATED) 6.6G (2.2G)	
CARB 20G	
FIBRE 1.5G	
CAL 186	

SUMMER COUSCOUS SALAD

PREP TIME: 3 MIN
COOK TIME: 12 MIN

280g couscous
500ml chicken or
  vegetable stock,
  simmering
2 garlic cloves, crushed
1 tbsp olive oil
1 tsp salt
1 tsp cinnamon
1 tsp cumin
1 tsp ground ginger
1 tsp turmeric
80g sultanas
1 cucumber, peeled,
  halved lengthwise,
  deseeded and diced
1 red pepper, diced
1 yellow pepper, diced
zest of 1 lemon
freshly ground pepper

FOR THE DRESSING
juice of 1 lemon
1 tbsp olive oil
½ tsp salt

This salad is based on a Dorie Greenspan recipe. It can be pulled together in no time at all: while the couscous is cooking, you can prepare all of the vegetables. It's a go-to salad in my kitchen and I especially like to eat it as a side with chicken or fish. It's also gorgeous with a dollop of hummus and served for lunch or a light dinner. Perfect for a meatless Monday!

Place the couscous in a large bowl. Place the chicken stock, garlic, olive oil, salt and spices in a large measuring jug and whisk until combined. Pour the stock over the couscous and stir to combine. Scatter the raisins over the couscous. Place a tea towel over the bowl and leave the couscous to cook for 10 minutes or according to the instructions on the package. Meanwhile, prepare the vegetables.

Fluff the couscous with a fork. Stir in the vegetables and lemon zest. Place all of the ingredients for the dressing in a jar with a lid and shake to combine. Pour the dressing over the couscous and toss well. Season with pepper and divide the salad between serving plates.

PROTEIN 9G	
FAT (SATURATED) 4.1G (0.7G)	
CARB 45G	
FIBRE 5.1G	
CAL 265	

TUNA & QUINOA SALAD

PREP TIME: 2 MIN
COOK TIME: 2 MIN
(ASSUMING YOU HAVE COOKED QUINOA)

2 small bowls of cooked
  quinoa
2 tbsp sundried tomato
  pesto
2 handfuls of green
  beans, sliced crossways
2 handfuls of salad leaves
160g tinned tuna,
  drained
a handful of basil leaves,
  torn

Quinoa was a staple in my kitchen long before it became a trendy ingredient. Ten years ago I had a list of the food shops in Ireland that stocked quinoa – it was not a long list! Nowadays, fortunately, quinoa can be easily found. Every week, I cook a big batch of quinoa and store it in the fridge. It's a delicious grain with a lot of health benefits. Use quinoa as a base for salads and you'll never run out of options. You can use tinned tuna or salmon in this salad. Either option will make a super-tasty and healthy lunch that's ready in no time at all.

Place the cooked quinoa and pesto in a large serving bowl and stir well to combine. Add the green beans and salad leaves and mix well. Scatter over the tuna and basil and serve.

PROTEIN 46G	
FAT (SATURATED) 22G (3G)	
CARB 30G	
FIBRE 6.9G	
CAL 516	

ROCKET, FENNEL & ORANGE SALAD

PREP TIME: 10 MIN
COOK TIME: 1 MIN

2 handfuls of rocket, washed and dried thoroughly
½ fennel, trimmed and cut into bite-sized pieces
1½ oranges, skin and outer pith removed, flesh cut into segments
juice of ½ orange
50g Wensleydale cheese with cranberries, crumbled

This salad sounds fancy but it is easy-peasy to make. The flavours combine beautifully and it looks so colourful on the plate. The rocket and orange provide a healthy dose of vitamin C, which will give your immune system a boost. I love to eat this salad with some barbecued meat or fish on a sunny summer's day.

Place the rocket, fennel and orange flesh in a large serving bowl and mix well. Drizzle over the orange juice. Crumble over the cheese and serve.

PROTEIN 8.4G

FAT (SATURATED) 8.3G (4.9G)

CARB 11G

FIBRE 3.6G

CAL 161

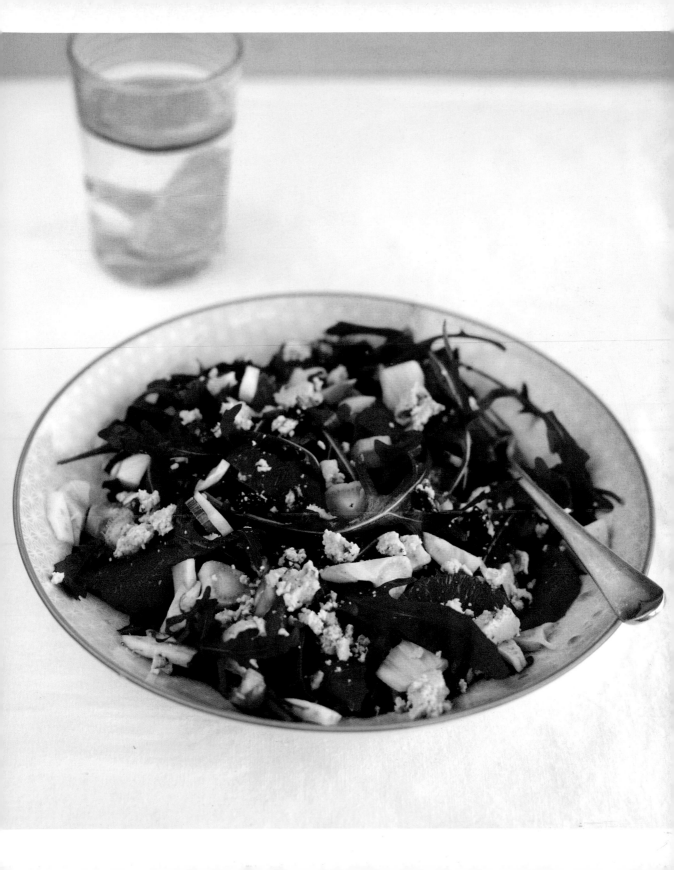

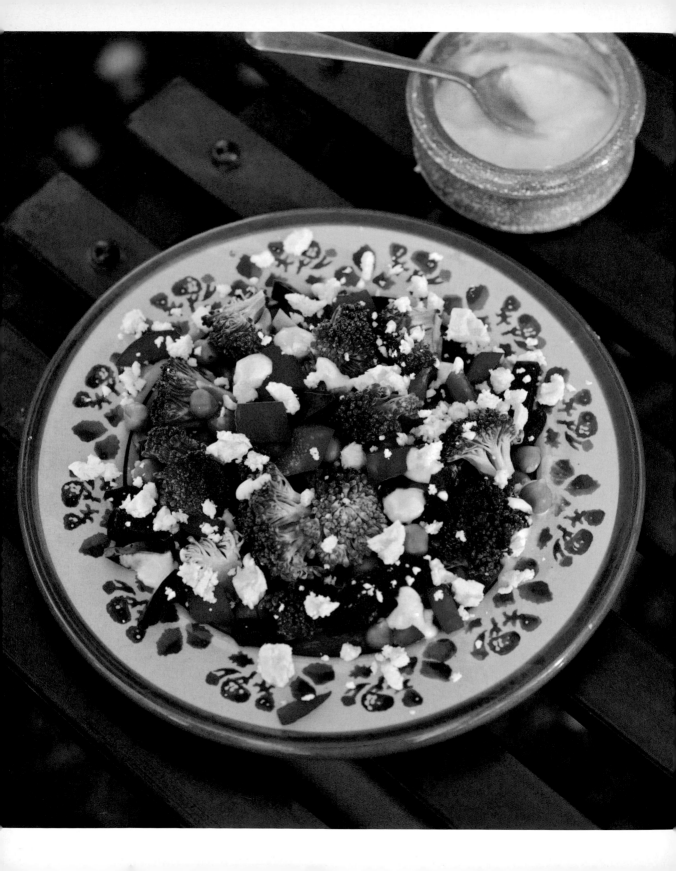

CRUNCHY BROCCOLI & FETA SALAD

PREP TIME: 10 MIN

400g broccoli florets, cut
    into bite-sized pieces
400g tin of chickpeas,
    drained and rinsed
2 peppers, deseeded and
    diced
75g feta, diced

FOR THE DRESSING

2 garlic cloves, crushed
4 tbsp natural yoghurt
1 tbsp lemon juice
salt and pepper

This is a tasty high-fibre salad. The raw broccoli and peppers have a lovely crunch that's offset by the feta, and the chickpeas pack in extra protein, complex carbohydrates and fibre. If you want to increase your carbohydrates, serve wholemeal pitta on the side. This is a salad that's easy enough to pull together in 10 minutes, but nice enough to serve to friends.

Place the broccoli, chickpeas, peppers and feta in a large serving bowl and mix well. Place all of the ingredients for the dressing in a small bowl and stir well. When you are ready to serve the salad, pour the dressing over it and toss well.

PROTEIN 17.7G
FAT (SATURATED) 9G (3.3G)
CARB 24G
FIBRE 9.6G
CAL 271

QUINOA SALAD WITH TOASTED NUTS & BLUE CHEESE

PREP TIME: 5 MIN (ASSUMING YOU HAVE COOKED QUINOA)
COOK TIME: 10 MIN

125g cooked quinoa
a handful of baby
  spinach
2 tbsp toasted nuts
  (almonds, pine nuts
  and cashews work well)
2 tbsp seeds (pumpkin
  and sunflower work
  well)
25g blue cheese,
  crumbled
a handful of blueberries
½ pomegranate, seeds
  only
a handful of mint leaves,
  chopped

FOR THE DRESSING
1 tbsp olive oil
1 tbsp natural yoghurt
juice of ½ lime
a pinch of sea salt

Since my fridge is never without a big batch of cooked quinoa, I tend to eat quinoa-based salads. I usually have a good stash of toasted nuts in my cupboard too. This means that I always have the basics at hand for interesting and nutritious lunches. Don't be put off by the blue cheese in this recipe. Even if you think you don't like it, you might be surprised at how well it complements the other flavours in this superfood salad.

Place the quinoa, spinach, nuts and seeds in a serving bowl and mix well.

Place all of the ingredients for the dressing in a jar with a lid and shake to combine. Pour this dressing over the quinoa salad and toss well. Crumble over the blue cheese. Scatter over the blueberries, pomegranate seeds and mint. The salad is ready to serve.

PROTEIN 11.2G	
FAT (SATURATED) 21G (4.5G)	
CARB 23G	
FIBRE 4.3G	
CAL 336	

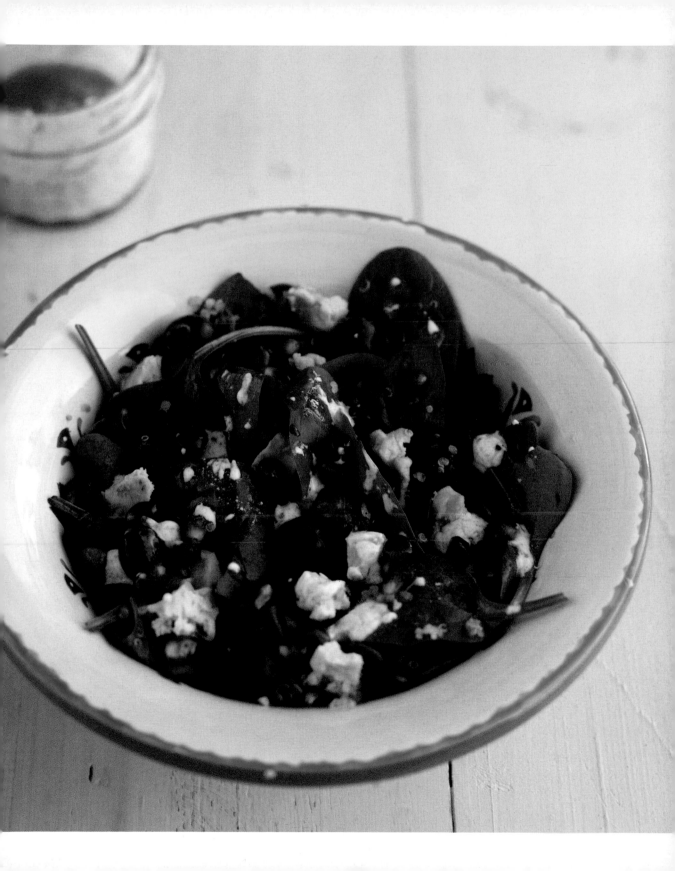

THREE-GRAIN SALAD

PREP TIME: 5 MIN (ASSUMING ALL PRE-COOKED INGREDIENTS ARE TO HAND)

100g brown rice, cooked and cooled (100g is the weight before cooking)

100g quinoa, cooked and cooled (100g is the weight before cooking)

100g wild rice, cooked and cooled (100g is the weight before cooking)

1 butternut squash, peeled, deseeded, cubed, roasted and cooled

3 roasted peppers (p. 141), sliced and cooled

1 pomegranate, seeds only

100g seeds (pumpkin and sunflower work well)

a handful of mint leaves, chopped

1 lemon, halved

Quinoa is not the only grain I eat for lunch. I love brown rice, wild rice and basmati too. I often purposely cook more rice than I need, so that I have leftovers to play with. If you're pre-cooking grains to be used in a cold salad, remember to cool the cooked grains as quickly as possible and store them in the fridge until you need them. It is true that making this Three-Grain Salad means being prepared. But if you can do a little planning and have all of the ingredients to hand, I promise it will be worth your while.

Store all of the cooled ingredients separately in the fridge until needed.

When you are ready to serve, toss the cooled ingredients together in a large bowl. Divide the salad between serving plates. Sprinkle over the seeds and mint. Squeeze over some lemon juice and serve without delay.

PROTEIN 12.1G	
FAT (SATURATED) 18.4G (2.4G)	
CARB 42G	
FIBRE 10.3G	
CAL 407	

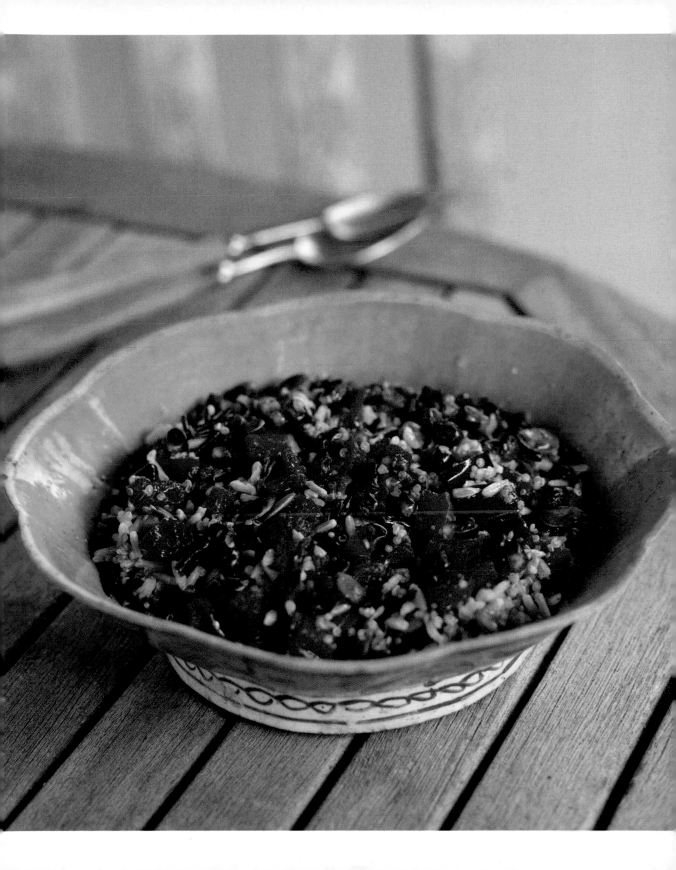

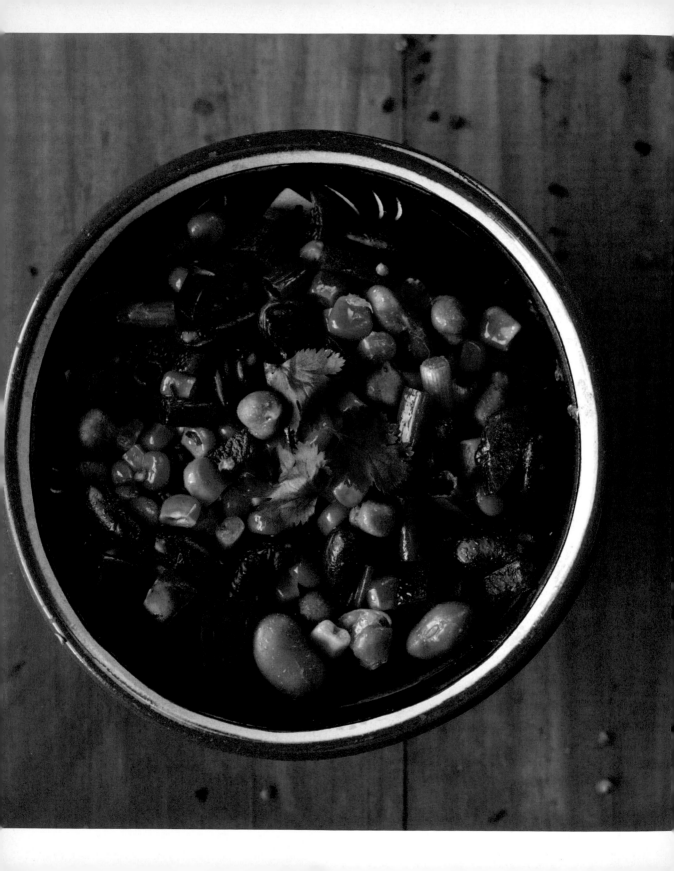

SERVES 2

THREE-BEAN SALAD

PREP TIME: 15 MIN

400g tin of mixed beans, drained and rinsed
80g tin of sweetcorn, drained and rinsed
3 scallions, finely sliced
1 red pepper, finely chopped
a handful of coriander leaves

FOR THE DRESSING
2 tbsp olive oil
1 tbsp agave syrup
1 tsp red wine vinegar
juice of 1 lime
a few drops of Tabasco sauce
¼ tsp chilli flakes
salt and pepper

It's a smart move to have plenty of tinned beans in your cupboard. Beans keep for ages, they're economical and they're complex foods that are rich in soluble fibre, polyphenols and folic acid. I rarely have time to soak and cook dried beans: good-quality tinned ones suit me just fine. This salad makes a filling and healthy lunch – and the Tabasco and chilli give it a nice spicy kick. It keeps really well, even with the dressing on, so it's an ideal workday lunch.

Place the beans, sweetcorn, scallions and red pepper in a large serving bowl and mix well. Place all of the ingredients for the dressing in a jar with a lid and shake to combine. Pour the dressing over the salad. Scatter over the coriander leaves and serve.

PROTEIN 17.2G	
FAT (SATURATED) 15.5G (2.2G)	
CARB 45G	
FIBRE 3.7G	
CAL 395	

TUNA PESTO PASTA

PREP TIME: 2 MIN
COOK TIME: 10 MIN

80g wholegrain pasta
112g tin of tuna in olive
  oil, drained
2 tbsp pesto (good-
  quality shop-bought
  works well)
a small handful of
  chopped scallions
2 tbsp grated Parmesan

This is a real student lunch – in the nicest possible sense! When I was in university, I was constantly going between the lecture hall, the track and the gym. Tuna Pesto Pasta was a lunch staple for me. And it still is nowadays: it always seems to set me up for a busy afternoon of work and running. The ingredients are simple and easy to find, and they combine into a nutritious lunch. The tuna is full of omega-3 goodness and the pasta will boost your energy for the afternoon ahead. This dish is delicious cooked fresh and served hot, but the leftovers are equally tasty as a cold pasta salad. A no-fuss, tasty lunch if ever there was one.

Cook the pasta according to the instructions on the package. Drain the pasta and return it to the pot. Stir in the tuna, pesto and scallions and heat through. Scrape the pasta into a warmed serving bowl. Sprinkle over the Parmesan and serve.

PROTEIN 52G

FAT (SATURATED) 39G (10.2G)

CARB 51G

FIBRE 8.4G

CAL 784

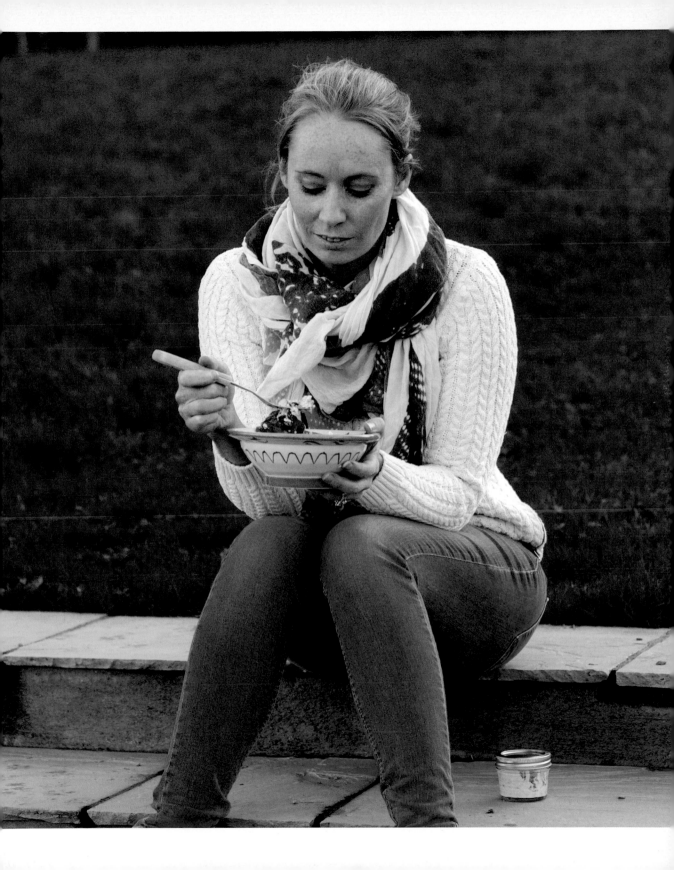

DINING *AL DESKO*

Bringing your own lunch to work is usually cheaper and nicer than grabbing something from a sandwich bar or eating out. These tips can be your starting point. Think of all the money that you can save and then spend on fancy training gear!

LOVE YOUR LEFTOVERS

Some meals just taste so good the following day that it would be a shame not to make extra and pack the leftovers for lunch. Try Chilli Bacon Beans (p. 35), Butternut and Bean Stew (p. 126), Chicken Tagine (p. 96) or Chilli con Carne (p. 76).

PACK IT UP

Pack your lunch the night before. Do it after dinner and the decision is already made for tomorrow's lunch!

HAVE A PREP DAY

If you have a few hours to spare in the week, such as on a Sunday evening, use this time to cook up a batch of recipes in preparation for the week ahead. You will be delighted later in the week when you are happily munching on an interesting lunch.

SNACK ATTACK

For those days when your lunch is just not inspiring, it's great if you can have a few snacks or extras on hand to throw in the lunchbox. Posh Nuts (p. 169) are a perfect way to spruce up an otherwise dull lunch.

SHARE THE LOAD

If you have a housemate or partner, make a deal with them that you will take turns in making lunch for both of you. It takes practically the same effort to make one lunch as two, so you might as well help each other out.

MIX-N-MATCH

Keep an open mind when you look in the fridge and don't be afraid to shake things up. I often have a work lunch that's a combination of leftovers from different meals, such as leftover stew and leftover salad. It sounds weird but it works.

GET EQUIPPED

Funky cooler bags, flasks and BPA-free plastic containers are easy to find. Buy one or two nice pieces of equipment and you're halfway there.

FRIDAY FEELING

Choose one day in the week for eating lunch out. Friday is my day for this. It gives me a great chance to get out of the office for an hour and socialize with work friends.

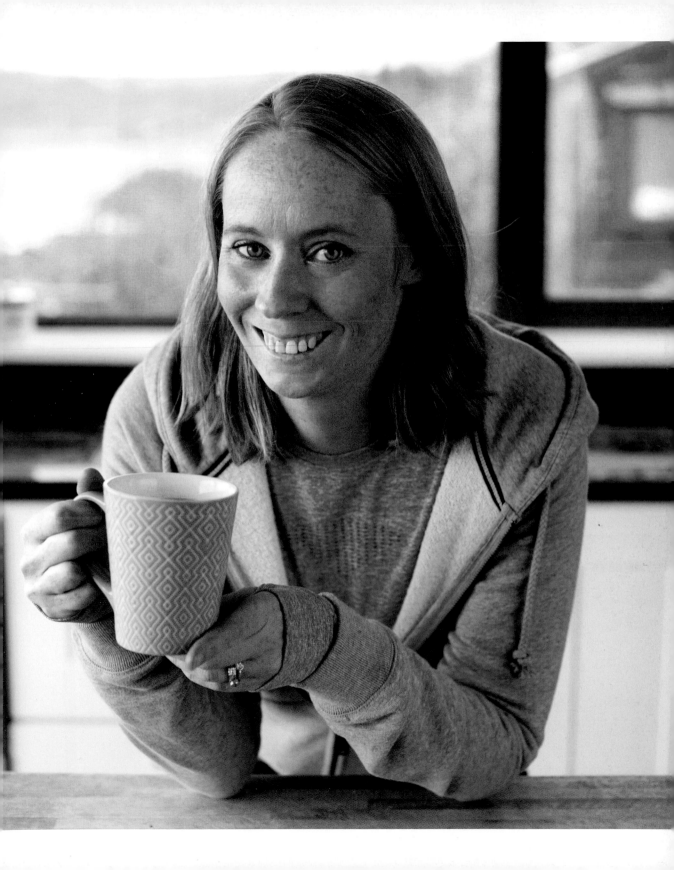

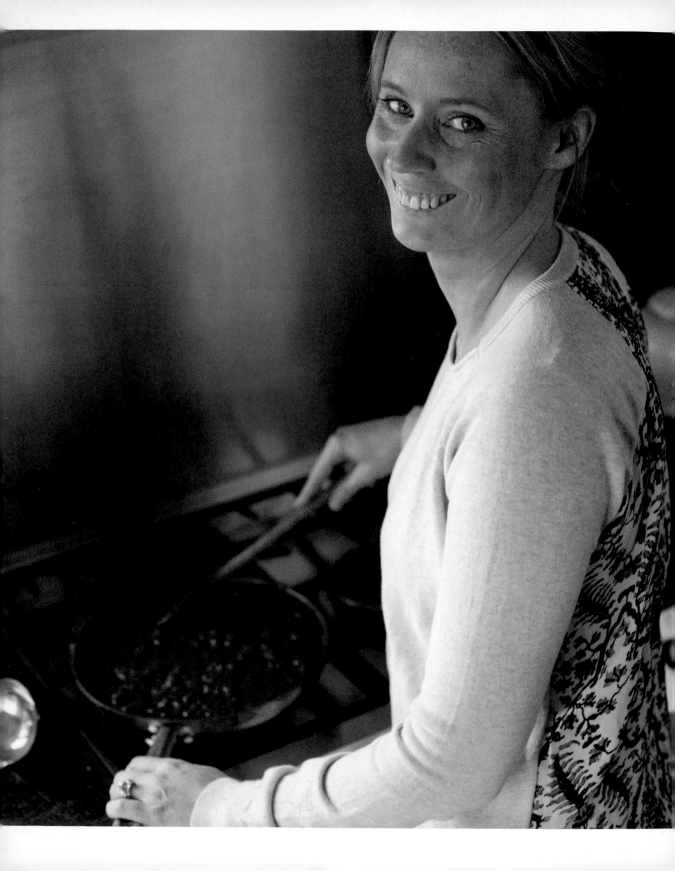

DINNER

FIT FOODIE CHILLI CON CARNE

EGGS-MEX

FIT FOODIE LASAGNE

MOROCCAN BEEF STEW

SPICY LAMB PITTA POCKET

LAID-BACK LAMB TAGINE

JOGGER'S CHICKEN STEW

CHICKEN TAGINE

SUPER-FAST STIR-FRY

CHICKEN, KALE & LEMONY RICE

LEMONY CHICKEN STEW

ONE-POT CHICKEN STEW

CHICKEN, PASTA & PEA BROTH

CHICKEN & KALE STIR-FRY

THAI-STYLE CHICKEN CURRY

TURKEY & TOMATO MEATBALLS

TURKEY CURRY

TURKEY STIR-FRY

FIT FOODIE FISH STEW

HONEY-SOY SALMON WITH NOODLES

EASY-PEASY SALMON BAKE

MEDITERRANEAN SALMON & SPAGHETTI

FIT FOODIE NUT ROAST

TOMATO & AUBERGINE BAKE

BUTTERNUT & BEAN STEW

FIT FOODIE CHILLI CON CARNE

**PREP TIME: 10 MIN
COOK TIME: 45 MIN**

coconut oil
2 onions, finely chopped
4 garlic cloves, crushed
1 chilli, finely chopped
2 tsp paprika
1¼ kg lean minced beef
2 × 400g tins of chopped
   tomatoes
a handful of cherry
   tomatoes, halved
500ml beef stock
5 tbsp tomato purée
400g tin of kidney beans,
   drained and rinsed
250g natural yoghurt
a handful of chives,
   chopped
salt and pepper
brown rice, to serve

I'm happy to eat chilli con carne at any time of year but I think it's particularly good in winter. It always gives my senses a wake-up call, especially if I've had a busy or tiring day. This recipe has a garlic and chilli kick, which should brighten up any dinnertime. Leftovers are portable and perfect for a workday lunch. The meat sauce freezes really well too, so it's a great recipe to make in big batches. If I had a whole rugby team over for dinner, this is what I would make!

Melt a tablespoon of coconut oil in a large pan over a medium heat. Add the onions and cook for 5 minutes, until softened. Add the garlic, chilli and paprika and cook for 5 minutes, stirring frequently. Melt a tablespoon of coconut oil in another large pan over a medium heat. Add the beef and cook for about 5 minutes, until golden brown. Use a slotted spoon to remove the cooked mince, discarding the fat in the pan.

Place the cooked mince into the pan with the onions. Add the chopped tomatoes, cherry tomatoes, stock and tomato purée and stir well. Simmer, uncovered, for 20 minutes. Stir in the kidney beans and cook for 5 minutes.

Meanwhile, mix the yoghurt and chives in a medium bowl and set aside. When you are ready to serve, season the chilli con carne to taste. Ladle it into warmed serving bowls and top each portion with a tablespoon of the yoghurt and chives. Serve with brown rice.

PROTEIN 78G

FAT (SATURATED) 31G (15.6G)

CARB 38G

FIBRE 9.3G

CAL 765

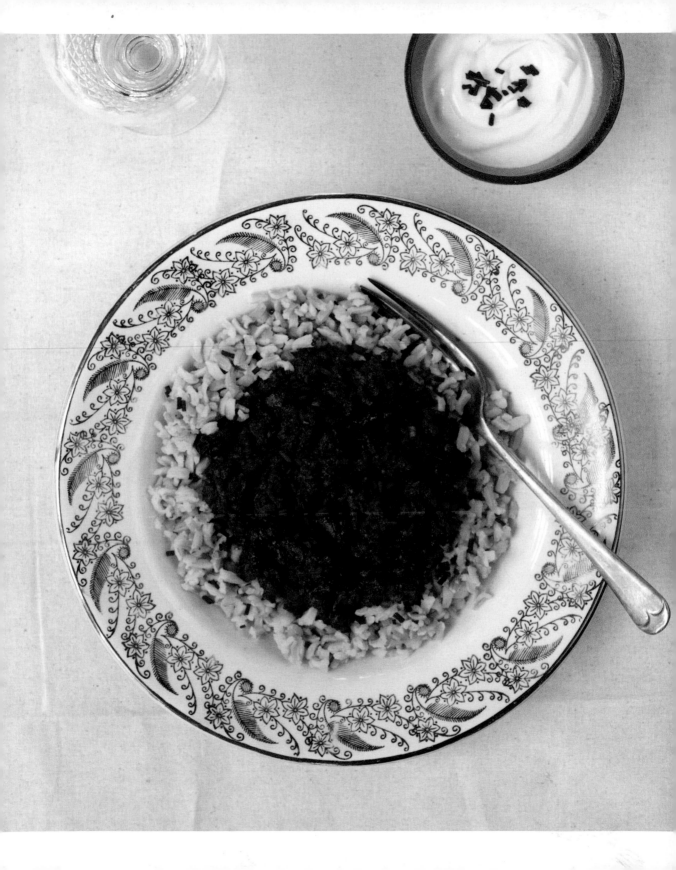

EGGS-MEX

PREP TIME: 5 MIN
COOK TIME: 25 MIN

2 tbsp coconut oil
1 onion, finely chopped
2 peppers, finely
  chopped
400g lean minced beef
2 tbsp fajita spice mix
400g tin of chopped
  tomatoes
3 eggs
50g Cheddar, grated
a handful of coriander
  leaves
3 tbsp natural yoghurt
3 wholemeal pittas,
  toasted (optional)

My mother-in-law, Sally, keeps hens. The birds have a spacious run and a view of the sea. I often joke that the birds are the most spoiled hens in Ireland. In return for the fancy accommodation, the hens produce a lot of eggs (seems like a fair deal to me). We regularly find ourselves with a glut of eggs and we have to be inventive in finding ways to use them up. This recipe came about when we had too many eggs and the coriander in our veggie patch was growing like a weed! The first time I made this recipe involved some wild experimentation – but it's become a recipe that's now very popular in our house.

Melt the coconut oil in a large pan over a medium heat. Add the onion and peppers and cook for 5 minutes, until softened. Stir in the mince and fajita spice. Cook for about 10 minutes, stirring often, until the beef is cooked through. Stir in the tomatoes and cook for 5 minutes. Use a ladle to create three shallow wells, each one about 5cm wide, in the mince. Crack one egg into each of the wells in the mince. (If you are an expert egg-cracker, just crack them straight into the wells. Otherwise, crack each egg in turn into a cup and then gently tip the egg from the cup into the well.) Reduce the heat to low and cover the pan with a lid. Leave the eggs to cook for about 4 minutes, until the white is set.

Remove the pan from the heat and sprinkle over the Cheddar. Divide the mince between warmed serving plates, ensuring that each person gets an egg. Sprinkle over the coriander. Serve with a dollop of natural yoghurt and toasted pitta on the side.

PROTEIN 38G	
FAT (SATURATED) 46G (27G)	
CARB 54G	
FIBRE 7.9G	
CAL 795	

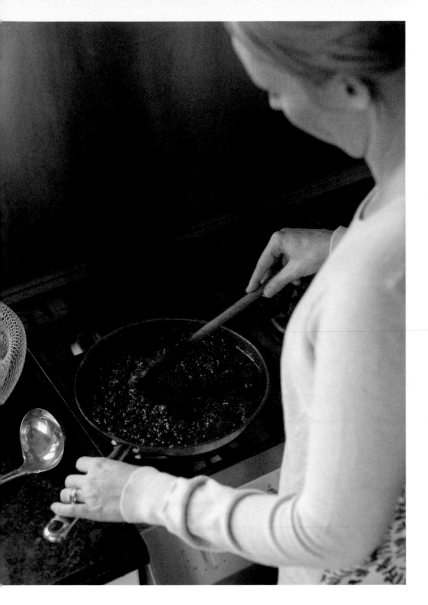
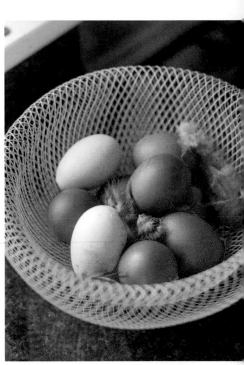
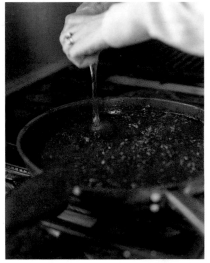
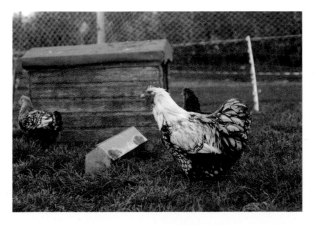

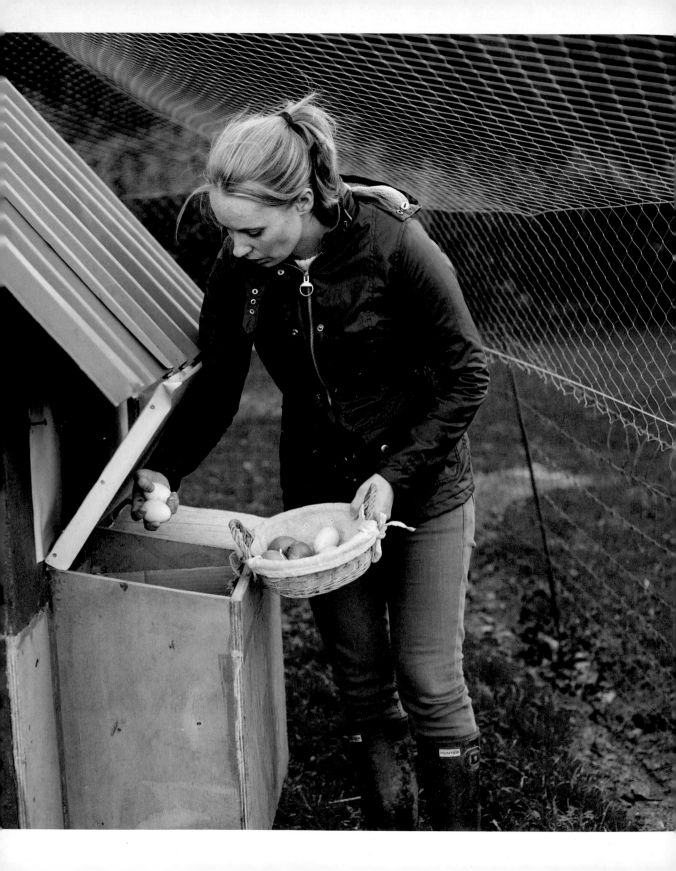

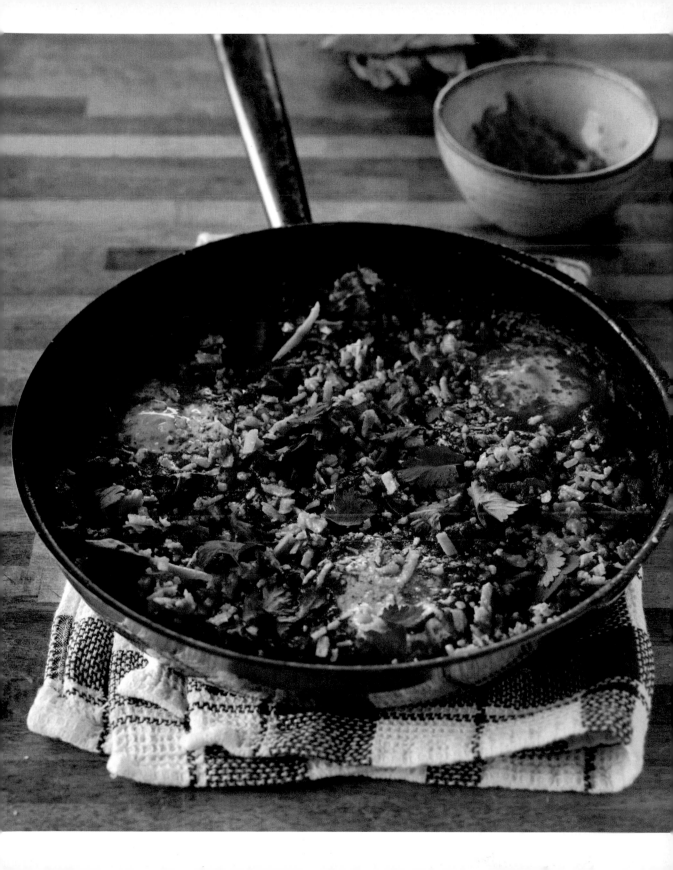

FIT FOODIE LASAGNE

Lasagne is a dish I regularly have as an indulgence if I'm out for dinner. At home, I make a leaner version: Fit Foodie Lasagne. I use only a little butter and cheese, and I use spelt flour instead of white flour – but it still tastes deliciously rich. Lasagne can be a bit of work but it's always worth the effort. I often make the Fit Foodie Tomato Sauce in advance, which means that the Fit Foodie Lasagne itself is no work at all. Consider making a double batch of this too. It's always good to have Fit Foodie Lasagne in your freezer: no matter how busy your week gets, you will still eat well.

**PREP TIME: 10 MIN
COOK TIME: 30 MIN
MAKES 500ML**

1 tbsp olive oil
1 carrot, peeled and finely chopped
1 celery stick, finely chopped
1 onion, finely chopped
1 red pepper, deseeded and diced
3 garlic cloves, crushed
400g tin of chopped tomatoes
1 tsp dried oregano
salt and pepper

FIT FOODIE TOMATO SAUCE

This sauce can be made well in advance and it can be used in stews and casseroles that call for chopped tomatoes. It makes a delicious pasta sauce too.

Heat the oil in a large pan over a medium heat. Add the carrot, celery, onion, pepper and garlic and cook for about 10 minutes, until softened. Add the tomatoes, oregano and 350ml of water and simmer, uncovered, for 20 minutes, stirring occasionally. Remove the pan from the heat. Purée the sauce with a hand blender until smooth. Season to taste. Place the cooled sauce in an airtight container and store in the fridge or freezer.

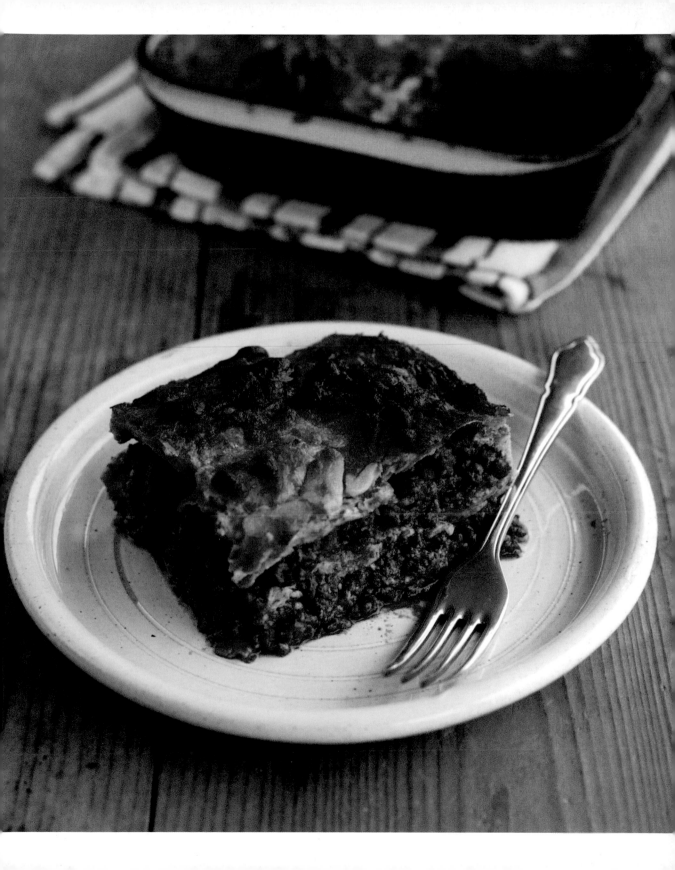

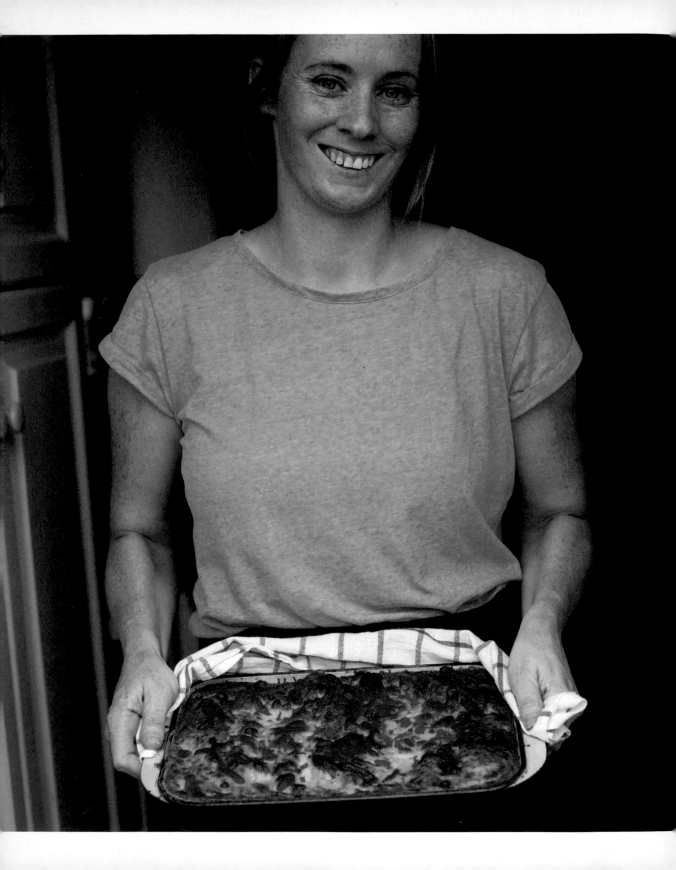

FIT FOODIE CHEESE SAUCE

PREP TIME: 5 MIN
COOK TIME: 15 MIN
MAKES 500ML

200ml milk
2 tbsp butter
1 bay leaf
½ tsp nutmeg
2 tbsp spelt flour
1 egg
1 tbsp natural yoghurt
25g Cheddar, grated
salt and pepper

This sauce is best made fresh and it's delicious with pasta, cauliflower or broccoli.

Place the milk, butter, bay leaf and nutmeg in a small pan. Slowly heat the milk and, just as it is about to reach boiling point and you see bubbles appearing around the edge of the pan, reduce to a low heat. Remove the bay leaf and add the flour. Use a whisk to blend the flour into the milk. Whisk for several minutes, until the sauce begins to thicken. Remove the pan from the heat. Add the egg and yoghurt and whisk until smooth. Whisk in the Cheddar and season to taste.

CREATING THE FIT FOODIE LASAGNE

PREP TIME: 5 MIN
COOK TIME: 35 MIN

2 tbsp olive oil
900g lean minced beef
1 quantity of Fit Foodie
  Tomato Sauce
a handful of basil leaves,
  chopped
150g wholewheat lasagne
  sheets (preferably fresh,
  but dried will work)
1 quantity of Fit Foodie
  Cheese Sauce

Preheat the oven to 180°C/350°F/gas 4. You will need a large lasagne dish.

Heat the oil in a large casserole over a medium heat. Add the mince and cook for about 10 minutes, until browned. Stir in the tomato sauce and basil and set aside while you assemble the lasagne.

Pour half of the mince into the lasagne dish. Top with a layer of lasagne sheets (about three sheets). Pour in the rest of the mince and top with a second layer of lasagne sheets. Pour the cheese sauce on top. Place the lasagne dish in the oven and cook for about 20 minutes, until golden and bubbling. Leave the cooked lasagne to stand for 5 minutes before dividing between warmed serving plates.

FIT FOODIE LASAGNE

PROTEIN 67G	
FAT (SATURATED) 41G (16.5G)	
CARB 26G	
FIBRE 3G	
CAL 749	

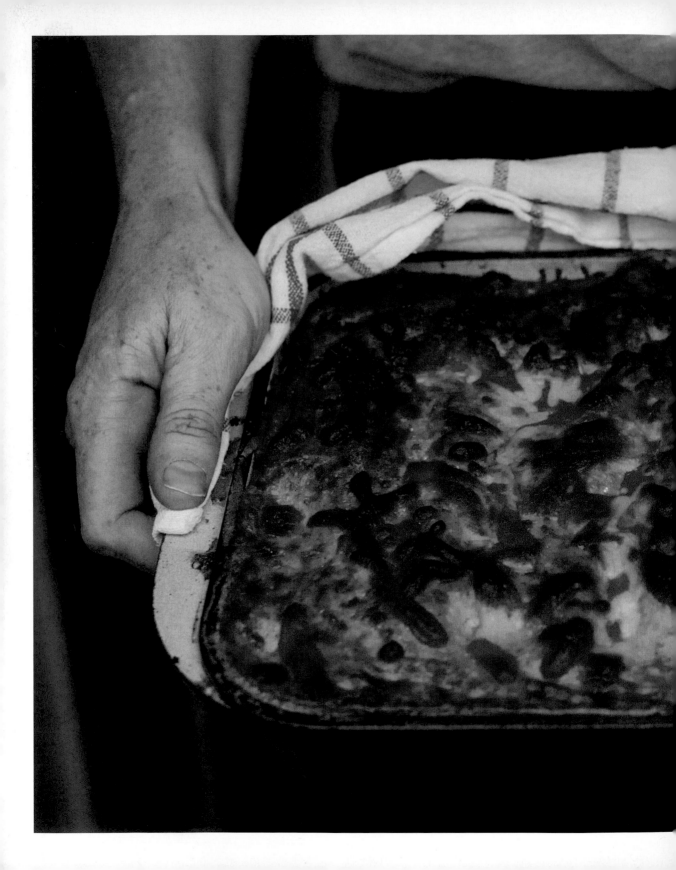

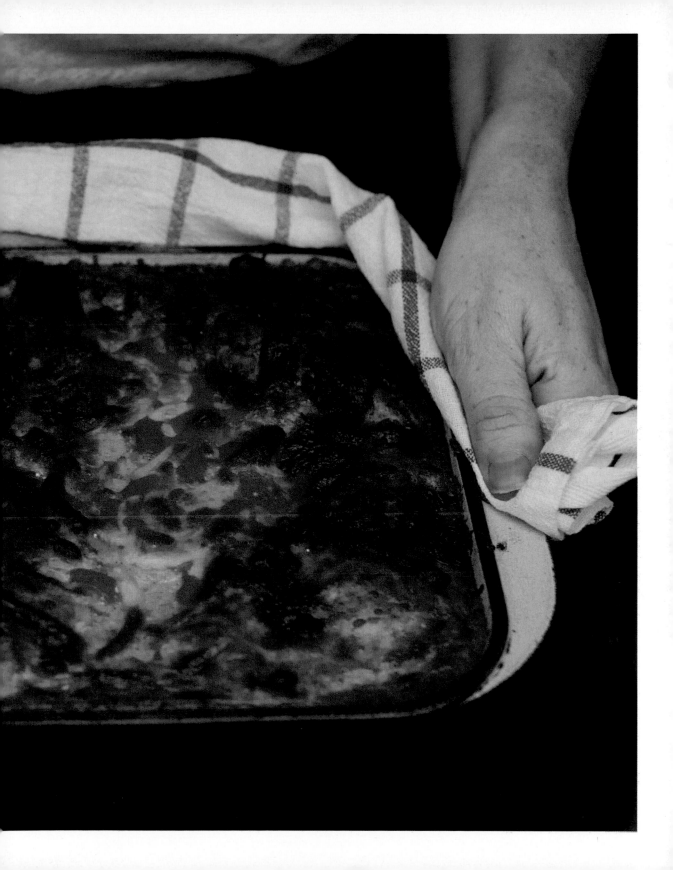

SERVES 4

MOROCCAN BEEF STEW

PREP TIME: 15 MIN
COOK TIME:
  1 HR 15 MIN

2 tbsp olive oil
600g lean stewing beef,
  cut into 3cm pieces
2 celery sticks, chopped
1 carrot, peeled and
  roughly chopped
1 onion, chopped
5 garlic cloves, crushed
a thumb-sized piece of
  fresh ginger, grated
1 tsp cinnamon
150ml red wine or beef
  stock
2 tbsp tomato purée
2 tbsp maple syrup
10 dried apricots, halved
a handful of mint leaves
brown rice, to serve

This is my go-to recipe when I want a beef stew with a bit of flair. I often cook a big batch of this stew on the weekend and then enjoy the leftovers midweek when time is tight. Even though this cooks in just an hour and a quarter, the beef comes out tender every time. If you want to stock up your freezer, make a double batch of this delicious stew.

Heat the oil in a large casserole over a medium heat. Brown the beef in batches and set aside on a plate. Reduce the heat and add the celery, carrot, onion, garlic, ginger and cinnamon. Cook, uncovered, for 5 minutes. Stir frequently and add a splash of water if the pan gets dry. Return the browned beef to the pot. Stir in the wine and simmer for 2–3 minutes, until the wine has reduced by half. Add 150ml of boiling water, tomato purée and maple syrup and stir well. Cover and simmer for 1 hour, stirring occasionally so that nothing sticks to the bottom of the pot.

Add the apricots and simmer, uncovered, for 15 minutes. Ladle the stew into warmed serving bowls and sprinkle over the mint. Serve with brown rice.

| PROTEIN 50G |
| FAT (SATURATED) 16G (4.4G) |
| CARB 19.2G |
| FIBRE 6.1G |
| CAL 465 |

SPICY LAMB PITTA POCKET

PREP TIME: 10 MIN
COOK TIME: 25 MIN

1 tbsp olive oil
1 onion, finely chopped
4 garlic cloves, crushed
½ chilli, finely chopped
1 tsp paprika
1 tsp turmeric
1 tbsp cumin
1 tbsp ground coriander
450g lamb mince
salt and pepper
4 tbsp natural yoghurt
½ cucumber, peeled,
  deseeded and diced
2 wholemeal pittas
2 tomatoes, chopped
a handful of fresh herbs,
  chopped (coriander,
  mint or parsley)

This is a recipe that keeps on giving: it makes a delicious hot dinner and the chilled leftovers are equally tasty. It's a great one to make if you know that you'll be dining *al desko* the following day, which I often am. Since the recipe serves two, you could eat it hot as a solo dinner and enjoy the chilled leftovers for your lunch the next day.

Heat the oil in a large pan over a medium heat. Add the onion and cook for about 5 minutes. Add the garlic, chilli and spices and cook for 4 minutes. Stir frequently and add a splash of water if the pan gets dry. Stir in the mince and cook for 15 minutes, until the lamb is cooked through. Season to taste.

Meanwhile, mix the yoghurt and cucumber in a small bowl.

When you are ready to serve, toast the pittas on both sides. Split open and stuff with the spicy mince. Top with the yoghurt, tomatoes and herbs and serve.

PROTEIN 68G

FAT (SATURATED) 38G (15.9G)

CARB 51G

FIBRE 7.5G

CAL 839

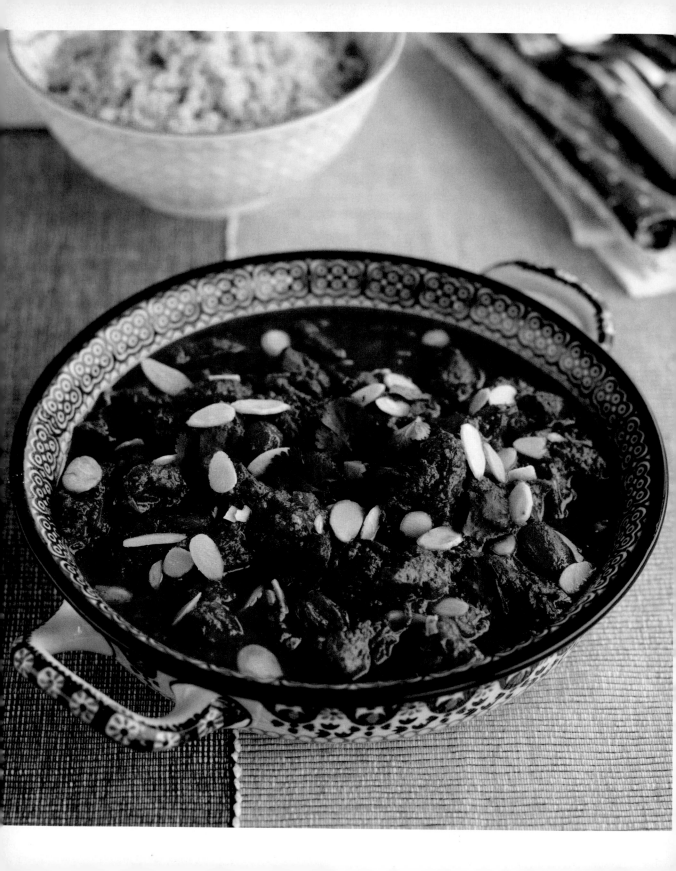

LAID-BACK LAMB TAGINE

**PREP TIME: 10 MIN
COOK TIME: 1 HR
15 MIN**

1kg shoulder of lamb,
  trimmed and diced into
  3cm pieces
1 tsp ground coriander
1 tsp cumin
1 tsp turmeric
2 tbsp ground almonds
2 tbsp honey
a handful of sultanas
400g tin of chopped
  tomatoes
1 tbsp olive oil
2 onions, finely chopped
5 garlic cloves, crushed
a thumb-sized piece of
  fresh ginger, grated
a handful of coriander
  leaves
a handful of flaked
  almonds
couscous, to serve

As a child, I went on a lamb boycott because I thought lambs were just too cute to eat. My mum continued to serve lamb for dinner but she told me it was beef, so I'd no problems eating that! I'm actually glad of my mum's trickery in this regard because, as a grown-up, lamb is one of my favourite meats to cook. Lamb is a good source of quality protein, iron and zinc, and it's really versatile. This tagine is such a laid-back dish to cook: you don't even need to brown the meat. The end result is delicious with the sweet honey and spices. A great meal to make for friends.

Place the lamb, spices, almonds, honey, sultanas and tomatoes in a large lidded casserole. Mix well and set aside.

Heat the oil in a frying pan and cook the onions, garlic and ginger for 5 minutes, until softened. Add the cooked onions to the lamb mixture in the casserole and stir well. Cover the casserole and place in the oven for 1 hour and 15 minutes, or until the lamb is tender.

Ladle the cooked tagine into warmed serving bowls. Sprinkle over the coriander and almonds. Serve with couscous.

PROTEIN 74G	
FAT (SATURATED) 32G (12.9G)	
CARB 24G	
FIBRE 2.8G	
CAL 688	

JOGGER'S CHICKEN STEW

PREP TIME: 5 MIN
COOK TIME: 2 HR
(INCLUDES THE
JOG!)

olive oil
4 large baking potatoes,
 washed, dried and
 pricked all over with
 a fork
salt and pepper
100g chorizo, sliced into
 1cm rounds
2 onions, finely sliced
12 cloves of garlic, peeled
4 tbsp flour
1 tbsp paprika
4 skinless chicken breast
 fillets
250ml chicken stock
250ml white wine
a sprig of rosemary (or a
 bouquet garni)
400g tin of kidney beans,
 drained and rinsed
 (mixed beans also
 work well)
500ml passata

PROTEIN 74G

FAT (SATURATED)
21G (3.6G)

CARB 117G

FIBRE 14.4G

CAL 990

I like to cook and eat well, but I like to pack a lot of other activities into my day too. I love those recipes that allow me to go off and do other things while dinner is cooking. This stew is one of those recipes. I take 30 minutes (tops!) to get it in the oven. Then I put on my running gear and head out jogging for an hour. When I get home, I check on the stew and stir in the last two ingredients for the final 30 minutes of cooking – which gives me just enough time to shower and set the table. It really is a dinner that cooks itself.

Preheat the oven to 180°C/350°F/gas 4. Rub a teaspoon of olive oil into the potatoes. Season the potatoes, wrap each one loosely in foil and set aside.

Heat a teaspoon of olive oil in a large lidded casserole over a medium heat. Add the chorizo, onions and garlic and cook for 5 minutes, stirring occasionally.

Meanwhile, mix the flour and paprika and spread them on a plate. Roll the chicken fillets on the plate to coat them with flour. Heat a tablespoon of olive oil in a frying pan over a medium heat. Fry the chicken fillets (in one batch) for 3 minutes on each side and set aside.

Pour the stock and wine into the casserole with the chorizo. Stir well. Add the chicken and rosemary and bring to the boil. Remove from the heat and cover the casserole with a lid. Place the casserole on a large baking tray along with the foil-covered potatoes. Lift the tray into the oven and cook for 1 hour.

Meanwhile, put on your runners and go for a jog!

After 1 hour, remove the casserole from the oven. Stir in the beans and passata. Return the casserole to the oven for 30 minutes. Ladle the stew into warmed serving bowls. Serve with the baked potatoes.

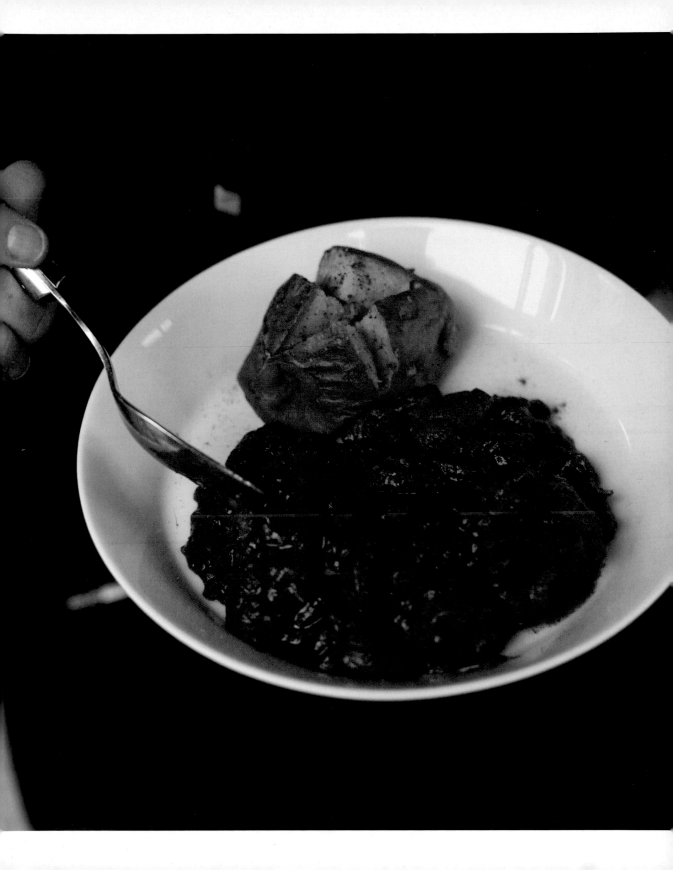

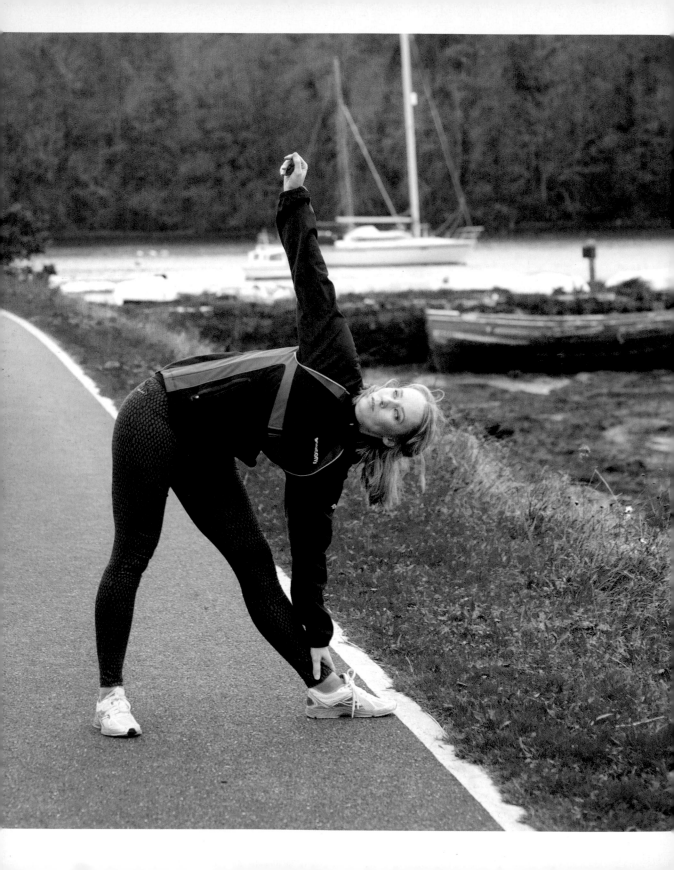

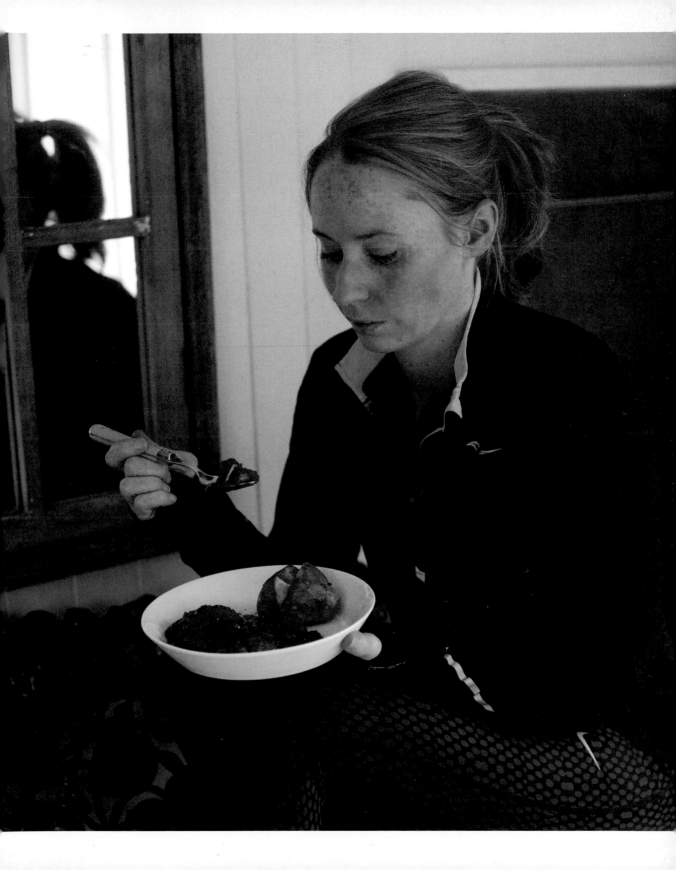

CHICKEN TAGINE

PREP TIME: 20 MIN
COOK TIME: 40 MIN

3 tbsp olive oil
1 onion, finely chopped
1 cinnamon stick, broken
   in half
3 skinless chicken breast
   fillets, cubed
½ butternut squash,
   peeled, deseeded and
   finely diced
1 red pepper, deseeded
   and diced
10 dried apricots,
   chopped
2 tsp ground ginger
250g couscous
500ml chicken stock
1 tbsp honey
a handful of flaked
   almonds
a handful of mint leaves,
   chopped

This tagine creates some serious aromas in the kitchen: cinnamon, ginger, apricots, honey and mint. There is no fuss in making this: it takes care of itself, really. This recipe makes three portions and it reheats beautifully the next day. If I make this for dinner, I'm always happy to eat the leftovers for lunch.

Heat the oil in a large pan over a medium heat. Add the onion and cinnamon stick and cook for 3 minutes. Stir frequently and add a splash of water if the pan gets dry. Add the chicken and cook for 5 minutes. Add the butternut, pepper, apricots and ginger and cook for 3 minutes. Stir in the couscous, chicken stock and honey. Reduce the heat and simmer for 15–20 minutes, until the couscous is cooked and has absorbed the liquid. Spoon the chicken tagine into warmed serving bowls. Sprinkle over the almonds and mint and serve.

PROTEIN 47G	
FAT (SATURATED) 17.8G (2.6G)	
CARB 86G	
FIBRE 15.6G	
CAL 731	

SUPER-FAST STIR-FRY

PREP TIME: 5 MIN
COOK TIME: 15 MIN

coconut oil
1 skinless chicken breast
  fillet, cubed
2 garlic cloves, crushed
a thumb-sized piece of
  fresh ginger, grated
½ onion, finely chopped
¼ red chilli, finely
  chopped
a handful of broccoli,
  broken into small florets
½ pepper, finely sliced
150g straight-to-wok rice
  noodles
1 tbsp soy sauce
juice of ½ lime
2 tbsp cashew nuts,
  chopped
a handful of mint leaves,
  chopped

It almost feels like cheating to write this up as a recipe. The truth is that it first came about when I arrived home from work one day absolutely starving and began to throw things into a pan in the hope that I would end up with a stir-fry that was edible. It was more than edible: it was delicious! Use the recipe below as a rough guide to quantities and flavours – but have fun, experiment and use whatever stir-fry vegetables are in your fridge. The straight-to-wok noodles make very light work of this delicious dinner.

Melt a tablespoon of coconut oil in a large pan over a medium heat. Add the chicken and cook for about 5 minutes, stirring occasionally, until the chicken is cooked through. Remove the chicken and set aside.

Add a teaspoon of coconut oil to the pan and increase the heat to medium-high. Add the garlic, ginger, onion and chilli and stir-fry for about 3 minutes. Add the broccoli and pepper and stir-fry for another 3 minutes. Return the cooked chicken to the pan and add the noodles, soy sauce and lime juice. Stir well and cook for 3 minutes or until the chicken and noodles are heated through. Spoon the stir-fry into a warmed serving bowl. Sprinkle over the cashew nuts and mint and serve.

PROTEIN 52G	
FAT (SATURATED) 43G (25G)	
CARB 29G	
FIBRE 3.8G	
CAL 727	

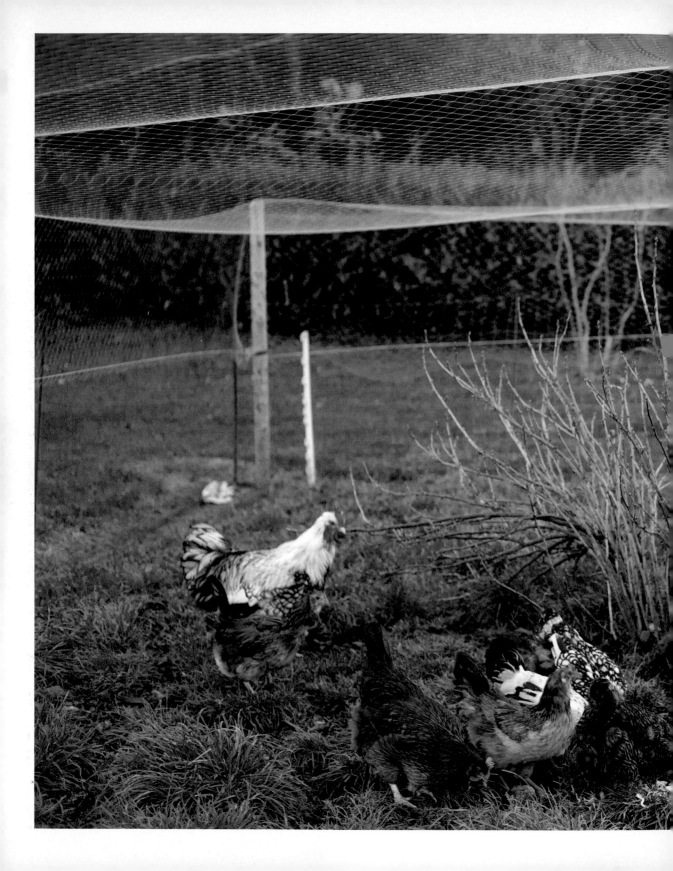

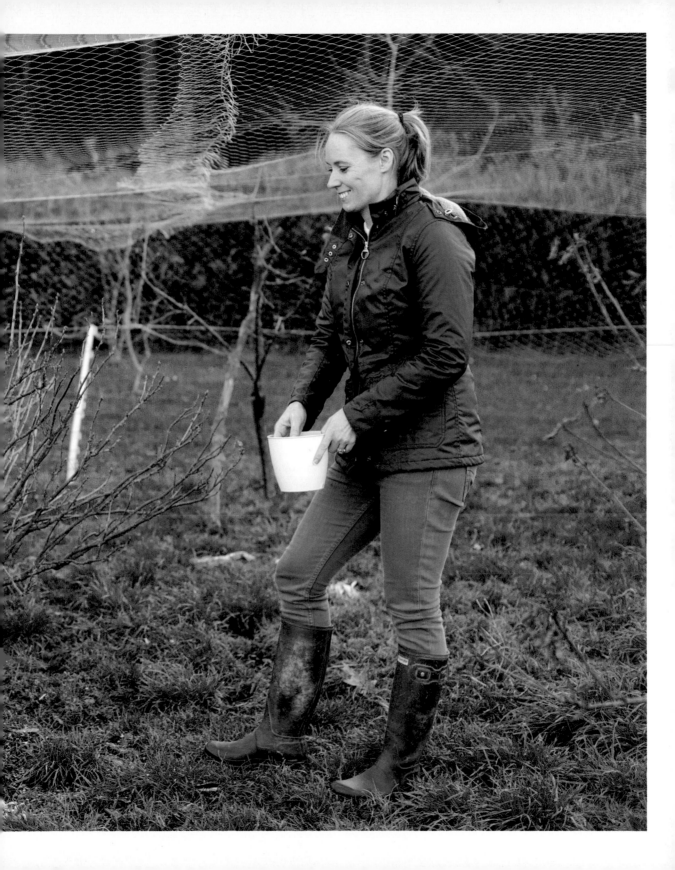

CHICKEN, KALE & LEMONY RICE

PREP TIME: 10 MIN
COOK TIME: 30 MIN

1 tbsp coconut oil
2 skinless chicken breast
   fillets, cubed
1 onion, chopped
a handful of kale leaves
2 garlic cloves, crushed
2 tbsp butter
1 tsp cumin
a pinch of ground saffron
   (optional)
juice of ½ lemon
125g brown rice
400ml chicken or
   vegetable stock

If you've never eaten kale before, consider giving it a go. Our grandmothers were eating it long before it became trendy! Kale contains considerable amounts of minerals, folates, carotenoids and prebiotic carbohydrates. This recipe is a great way to combine kale with lots of other healthy ingredients. It's the ultimate low-maintenance, one-pot midweek dinner.

Melt the coconut oil in a large casserole over a medium heat. Add the chicken and cook for 5 minutes or until cooked through. Remove the chicken and set aside.

Reduce the heat, add the onion and cook for 3 minutes. Add the kale, garlic, butter, cumin, saffron and lemon juice. Stir well and simmer, covered, for 5 minutes. Add the brown rice and stock and stir well. Cover the pot and simmer for 15 minutes, until the rice is just tender. Return the chicken to the casserole and cover the pot. Cook for 5 minutes, until the rice and chicken are heated through. Spoon the rice into warmed serving bowls.

PROTEIN 44G	
FAT (SATURATED) 22G (13.6G)	
CARB 51G	
FIBRE 2.5G	
CAL 579	

LEMONY CHICKEN STEW

**PREP TIME: 15 MIN
COOK TIME: 50 MIN**

1 tbsp coconut oil
2 onions, finely chopped
6 garlic cloves, crushed
a thumb-sized piece of
   fresh ginger, grated
1 tsp cinnamon
1 tsp cumin seeds
½ tsp paprika
4 skinless chicken breast
   fillets, cubed
2 peppers, deseeded and
   diced
10 dried apricots, halved
10 stoned green olives,
   halved
1 lemon, cut into wedges
½ courgette, chopped
300ml chicken stock
salt and pepper
a handful of mint leaves,
   chopped
brown rice, to serve

This stew brings back memories of being in Spain at the height of summer for a race on the international circuit. I ate the most delicious lemony chicken stew at lunchtime before I headed to the track. I tried to recreate the stew in my own kitchen as soon as I was back in Ireland. Whenever I feel a head cold coming on, I reach for this lemony stew!

Melt the coconut oil in a large casserole over a medium heat. Add the onions and cook for 5 minutes, until softened. Add the garlic and ginger and cook for 3 minutes. Add the cinnamon, cumin seeds and paprika and cook for 2 minutes. Stir frequently and add a splash of water if the pan gets dry. Add the chicken and cook for 5 minutes. Stir in the peppers, apricots, olives, lemon, courgette and stock. Reduce the heat and simmer, covered, for 30 minutes or until the chicken is cooked through and the vegetables are tender. When you are ready to serve, season to taste. Ladle the stew into warmed serving bowls and sprinkle over the mint. Serve with brown rice.

PROTEIN	39G
FAT (SATURATED)	10.1G (6.6G)
CARB	21G
FIBRE	8.2G
CAL	349

ONE-POT CHICKEN STEW

PREP TIME: 10 MIN
COOK TIME:
1 HR 30 MIN

2 tbsp butter
3 celery sticks, chopped
1 onion, finely chopped
1 tbsp fresh thyme leaves
4 chicken legs
4 garlic cloves, crushed
a glass of white wine
2 carrots, peeled and
   roughly chopped
400g tin of chopped
   tomatoes
salt and pepper
baby potatoes, to serve

I'm calling this a one-pot stew, even though I suggest cooking baby potatoes to serve on the side but . . . bear with me! The stew itself is done in one big pot: very little hassle or washing-up. While the stew serves four people, the leftovers reheat well – so consider making it even if it's just for one or two people. I use chicken legs in this stew because they're economical and they add a lot of flavour. If you want extra indulgence, top the baby potatoes with a knob of butter and a handful of chopped scallions.

Melt the butter in a very large casserole over a medium heat. Add the celery, onion and thyme and cook for 5 minutes. Place the chicken legs skin-side down in the pan and cook for 5 minutes, until the skin is browned. Add the garlic and cook for 2 minutes. Pour in the wine and cook on a high heat for 2 minutes, until the wine reduces. Reduce the heat and stir in the carrots and tomatoes. Simmer, uncovered, for 40 minutes.

Stir 200ml of water into the pan and turn the chicken legs so that they are skin-side up. Simmer, uncovered, for another 40 minutes.

Meanwhile, boil the potatoes in salted water for 10–15 minutes, until tender. When the chicken is cooked through and the vegetables are tender, season to taste. Ladle the stew into warmed serving bowls and serve with the baby potatoes.

PROTEIN 26G	
FAT (SATURATED) 25G (5.7G)	
CARB 32G	
FIBRE 6G	
CAL 468	

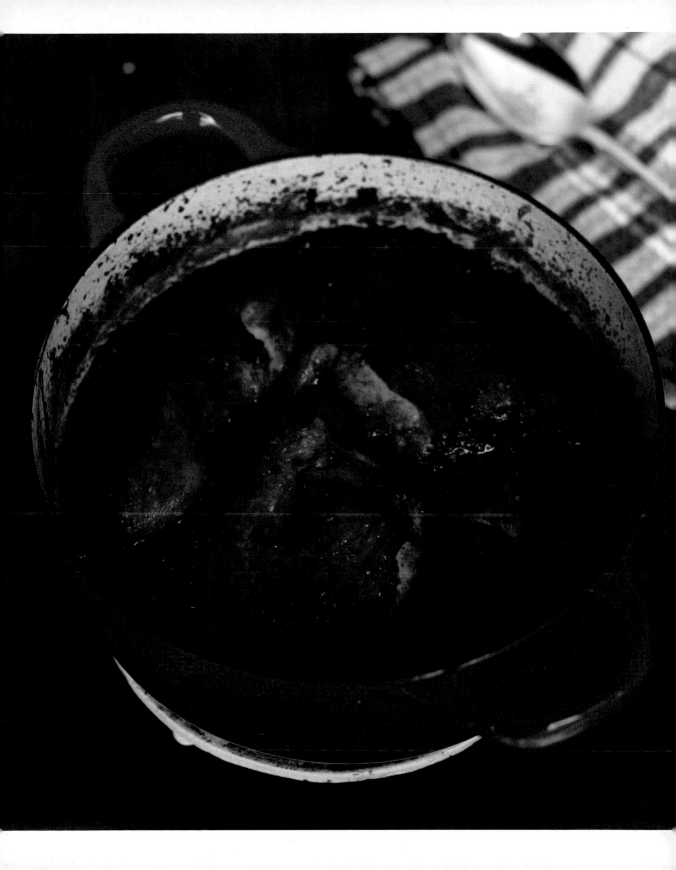

CHICKEN, PASTA & PEA BROTH

PREP TIME: 5 MIN
COOK TIME: 15 MIN

1 tbsp olive oil
2 skinless chicken breast
  fillets, finely sliced
100g spelt pasta
500ml chicken stock
50g frozen peas
a handful of chopped
  scallions
a handful of basil leaves,
  chopped

This is one of the quickest evening meals you could make. I'll reach for this midweek when I come home tired, maybe after an evening workout, and I want something simple but soothing. It's a really adaptable recipe, so don't be afraid to experiment. Try adding a little smoked bacon and parsley or thyme. The choices are endless with this one!

Heat the oil in a medium pan over a medium-high heat. Cook the chicken for 5 minutes or until cooked through. Drain the cooked chicken and set aside.

Meanwhile, cook the pasta according to the instructions on the package, but using chicken stock instead of water. Do not drain the pasta. Leave the cooked pasta and chicken stock to simmer together in the pan. Add in the cooked chicken, frozen peas and scallions and bring to the boil. Cook for about 3 minutes, until the chicken and vegetables are heated through.

Divide between warmed serving bowls. Sprinkle over the basil leaves and serve.

PROTEIN 66G	
FAT (SATURATED) 13.3G (2.7G)	
CARB 35G	
FIBRE 5.2G	
CAL 536	

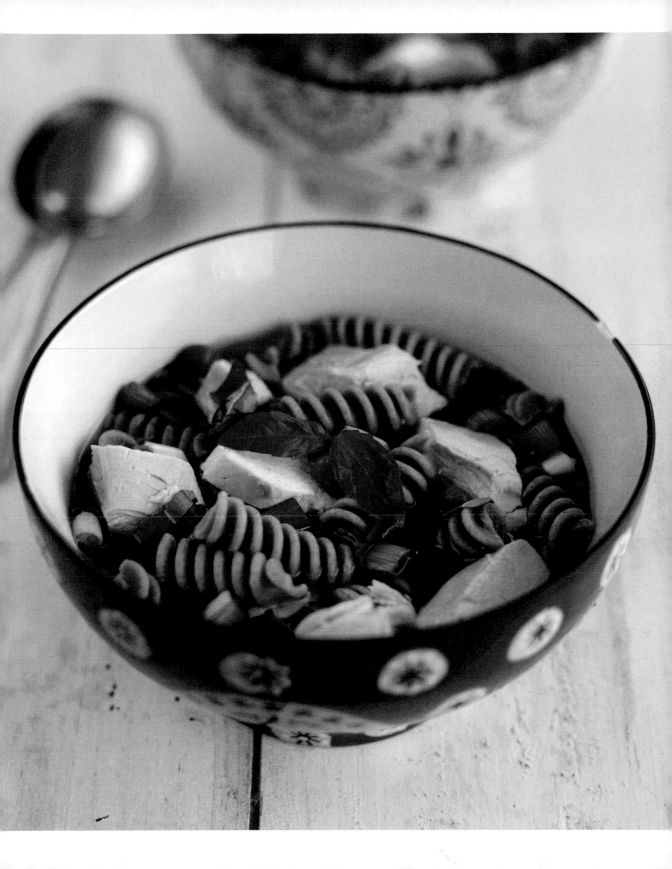

CHICKEN & KALE STIR-FRY

PREP TIME: 10 MIN
COOK TIME: 20 MIN

olive oil
2 skinless chicken
  breast fillets, sliced into
  medium strips
a handful of kale leaves
1 onion, finely sliced
2 garlic cloves, crushed
1 chilli, finely chopped
1 tsp grated fresh ginger
150g straight-to-wok
  noodles
100g cashew nuts
2 tbsp soy sauce
1 tbsp white rice vinegar
  (optional)
juice of 1 lime
a handful of mint leaves,
  chopped

This recipe is not a list of strict instructions. Just use it as a guideline and play around with the ingredients. If you don't have chicken, use turkey instead. If you don't have kale, use spinach. And if you have stir-fry vegetables that you want to use up, throw them in too. You'll have a delicious dinner in minutes.

Heat a tablespoon of olive oil in a large pan over a medium heat. Add the chicken and stir-fry for about 5 minutes, until the chicken is cooked through. Remove the chicken and set aside.

Place 250ml of water in a medium saucepan and bring to the boil. Add the kale and cook, covered, for about 5 minutes, stirring occasionally. Drain and set aside.

Meanwhile, heat a tablespoon of olive oil in a large pan over a medium-high heat. Add the onion and stir-fry for 2 minutes. Add the garlic, chilli and ginger and stir-fry for 2 minutes. Add the cooked kale, noodles, cashew nuts, soy sauce, rice vinegar and lime juice. Return the chicken to the pan and stir-fry until the chicken and noodles are heated through.

Divide the stir-fry between warmed serving bowls. Sprinkle over the mint and serve.

PROTEIN 60G
FAT (SATURATED) 32G (4.8G)
CARB 22G
FIBRE 3.2G
CAL 624

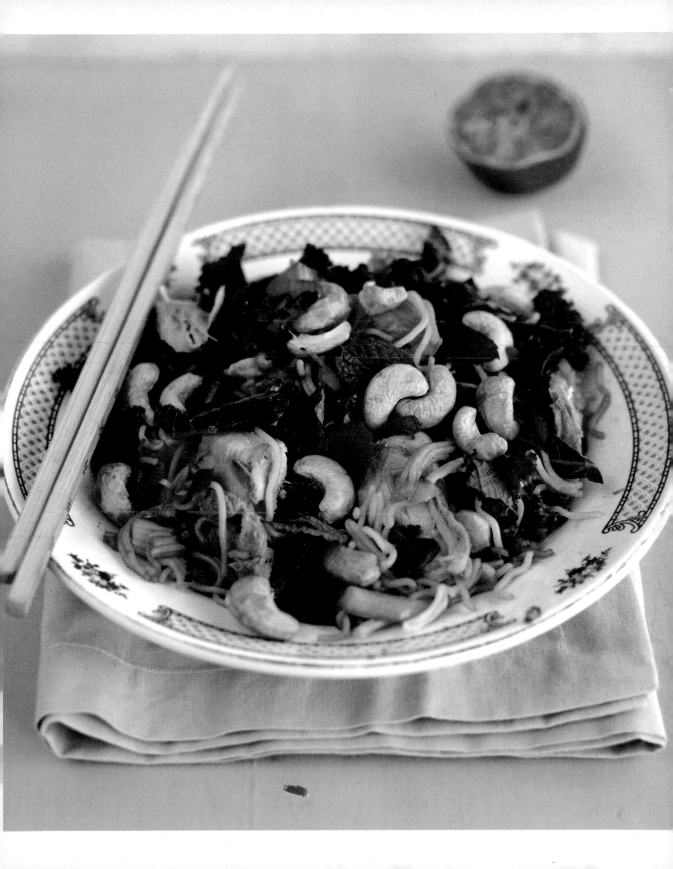

SERVES 6

THAI-STYLE CHICKEN CURRY

PREP TIME: 20 MIN (INCLUDES MARINATING)
COOK TIME: 15 MIN

5 skinless chicken breast fillets, cubed
1 tbsp coconut oil
3 red peppers, deseeded and cubed
1 onion, finely chopped
3 garlic cloves, crushed
300ml coconut milk
5 tbsp natural yoghurt
2 tsp cinnamon
2 tsp cumin
2 tsp turmeric
250g brown rice

FOR THE MARINADE
2 tbsp apple juice
2 tbsp soy sauce
1 tbsp ground almonds
2 tsp sesame oil

The peppers, onion and garlic add nutrition to this curry. I use garlic and onions wherever I can in cooking: they create a brilliant taste-base and they are also packed with prebiotics, which are vital in an athlete's diet. Of course, it's tender meat that really makes a good curry – and the marinade in this curry takes care of that.

Place the chicken in a medium bowl. Place all of the ingredients for the marinade in a jar with a lid and shake to combine. Pour the marinade over the chicken. Leave the chicken to marinate for 20 minutes while you prepare the rest of the ingredients.

Melt the coconut oil in a large pan over a medium heat. Add the peppers, onion and garlic. Cook for about 5 minutes, until softened. Stir in the coconut milk, yoghurt and spices. Add the marinated chicken to the pan. Simmer, uncovered, for 10 minutes or until the chicken is cooked through.

Meanwhile, cook the rice according to the instructions on the package.

Spoon the cooked rice into warmed serving bowls, making a well in the centre. Ladle the curry on top and serve.

PROTEIN	35G
FAT (SATURATED)	17.1G (9.5G)
CARB	26G
FIBRE	3.7G
CAL	405

SERVES 4

TURKEY & TOMATO MEATBALLS

PREP TIME: 10 MIN
COOK TIME: 40 MIN

2 tbsp olive oil
1 onion, finely chopped
1 carrot, finely chopped
1 fennel bulb, trimmed
  and finely sliced
4 garlic cloves, crushed
½ chilli, finely chopped
2 × 400g tins of chopped
  tomatoes
600g wholewheat or
  spelt spaghetti
a handful of herbs,
  chopped (parsley,
  coriander and dill
  work well)

FOR THE MEATBALLS
500g turkey mince
5 tbsp porridge oats
3 garlic cloves, crushed
1 egg
salt and pepper

Since turkey is a lean meat, it's often recommended to people when they need to trim down a bit. So I guess we should all make friends with turkey, right? The oats give a lovely texture to these turkey meatballs and pack in a bit of extra nutrition too.

Heat the oil in a large pan over a medium heat. Add the onion and cook for 4 minutes, until softened. Add the carrot, fennel, garlic and chilli and cook for about 6 minutes, until softened. Stir frequently and add a splash of water if the pan gets dry. Stir in the tomatoes and leave the sauce to simmer, uncovered, while you prepare the meatballs.

Place all of the ingredients for the meatballs in a large bowl and mix thoroughly with a spatula. Using wet hands, roll the mixture into 20 small meatballs. Wash your hands thoroughly. Gently stir the meatballs into the tomato sauce and cook, uncovered, for 15 minutes or until the meatballs are cooked through.

Meanwhile, cook the spaghetti according to the instructions on the package. Divide the cooked spaghetti between warmed serving bowls. Ladle the meatballs and tomato sauce on top. Sprinkle over the herbs and serve.

PROTEIN 49G	
FAT (SATURATED) 19.1G (4.2G)	
CARB 52G	
FIBRE 11G	
CAL 605	

TURKEY CURRY

PREP TIME: 10 MIN
COOK TIME: 50 MIN

1 tbsp olive oil
1 onion, finely chopped
2 tbsp medium curry
  powder
1 tbsp garam masala
1 tsp ground coriander
1 tsp cumin seeds
500g turkey breast,
  cubed
a thumb-sized piece of
  fresh ginger, grated
400ml tin of coconut
  milk
200g tin of chopped
  tomatoes
2 tbsp ground almonds
1 banana, peeled and
  sliced
brown rice, to serve

Turkey is well suited to curries and it makes a nice change from using chicken. Turkey is a lean meat and a brilliant source of protein – it's economical too. I love fruit in a curry and I think banana gives a special sweetness and texture in this dish. Of course, you can leave out the banana if you're not a fruity-curry kind of person. If you have any Mango Salsa (p. 146) to hand, it will add extra zing to this curry. Turkey Curry freezes and reheats really well – and the leftovers taste amazing.

Heat the oil in a large pan over a medium heat. Add the onion and spices and cook for 5 minutes, stirring frequently. Add the turkey and ginger and cook for 2 minutes. Stir in the coconut milk, tomatoes and almonds. Simmer, uncovered, for 40 minutes. (If you want a thicker sauce, you can cook this for up to 20 minutes longer, stirring frequently.)

Just before serving, stir the banana slices into the curry. Ladle the curry into warmed serving bowls and serve with brown rice.

PROTEIN 96G	
FAT (SATURATED) 41G (16.3G)	
CARB 29G	
FIBRE 8.1G	
CAL 887	

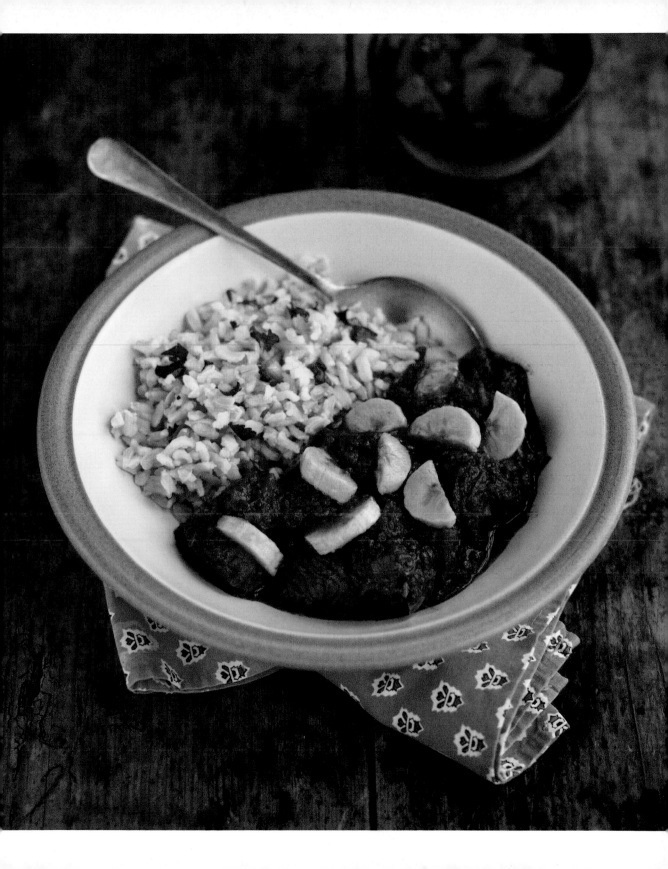

TURKEY STIR-FRY

PREP TIME: 5 MIN
COOK TIME: 15 MIN

2 tbsp coconut oil
1 onion, finely sliced
1 chilli, finely chopped
4 garlic cloves, crushed
a thumb-sized piece of
   fresh ginger, grated
a handful of broccoli,
   broken into small
   florets
1 carrot, peeled and cut
   into matchsticks
1 pepper, finely sliced
400g turkey mince
3 tbsp soy sauce
1 tbsp fish sauce
125g brown rice
a handful of basil leaves

Turkey is not just for Christmas! This recipe is quick to prepare and makes a tasty midweek dinner. It might seem strange to put minced meat into a stir-fry but it actually works really well with turkey because the smaller pieces of meat soak up all of the heat and flavours of chilli, ginger, garlic and soy sauce. This is another recipe where you don't have to stick rigidly to the ingredients list. Just use it as a guide and don't be afraid to experiment with the contents of your fridge.

Melt the coconut oil in a large pan over a medium-high heat. Add the onion, chilli, garlic and ginger and stir-fry for about 3 minutes. Add the broccoli, carrot and pepper and stir-fry for another 3 minutes. Add the turkey mince, soy sauce and fish sauce and stir-fry for 8 minutes or until the turkey is cooked through.

Meanwhile, cook the rice according to the instructions on the package.

Spoon the cooked rice into warmed serving bowls. Spoon the stir-fry on top. Before serving, tear the basil leaves and scatter them over the stir-fry.

PROTEIN 65G	
FAT (SATURATED) 42G (28G)	
CARB 61G	
FIBRE 5.9G	
CAL 896	

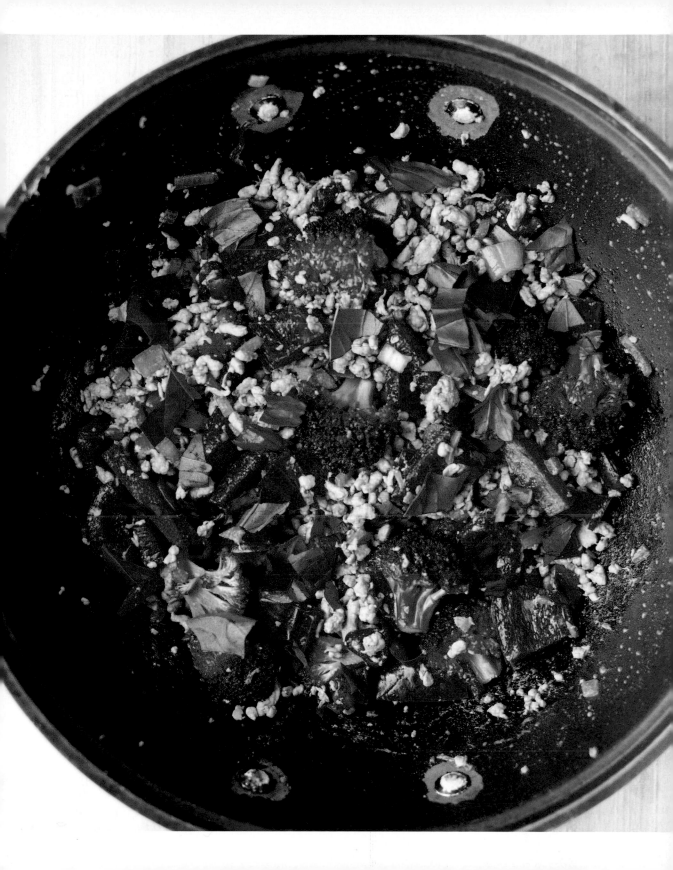

FIT FOODIE FISH STEW

**PREP TIME: 10 MIN
COOK TIME: 45 MIN**

2 tbsp olive oil
1 onion, chopped
4 tomatoes, roughly
  chopped
2 celery sticks, chopped
5 garlic cloves, crushed
zest and juice of ½
  lemon
12 baby potatoes, washed
  and halved
300ml vegetable or fish
  stock
600g mixed fresh
  fish fillets, cut into
  5cm pieces (ask your
  fishmonger)
white pepper
2 tbsp grated Parmesan
4 tbsp chopped
  coriander
4 tbsp chopped dill

I eat fish for dinner about three times a week. When I'm training hard, eating fish helps my muscles to recover. Fish is serious 'brain food' too – and since I pack a lot into my week, I figure I should give my brain all the help it can get!

There's no reason not to give fish a go, especially with recipes like this one. The tomato sauce keeps things light but full of flavour. And the whole thing is done in one pot. Yes, you'll have to make the effort to buy some nice fish; but you'll have practically no washing-up after dinner. Sounds like a nice trade-off to me.

Preheat the oven to 180°C/350°F/gas 4. Heat the olive oil in a large casserole over a medium heat. Add the onion and cook for 2 minutes. Stir in the tomatoes and cook for 3 minutes. Add the celery, garlic, lemon zest and juice and cook for 10 minutes, stirring frequently. Add the potatoes and stock and bring to the boil. Reduce the heat and simmer, uncovered, for 10 minutes. Add the fish and simmer for 10–15 minutes, until the fish is cooked through.

Remove the casserole from the heat and season the stew with white pepper. Sprinkle over the Parmesan and place the casserole in the oven for 5 minutes to create a crispy topping. Ladle the stew into warmed serving bowls. Sprinkle over the herbs and serve.

PROTEIN 35G	
FAT (SATURATED) 14.1G (3.5G)	
CARB 28G	
FIBRE 6.8G	
CAL 396	

HONEY-SOY SALMON WITH NOODLES

PREP TIME: 5 MIN
COOK TIME: 15 MIN

2 × 100g salmon fillets, skinned
1 tbsp butter
1 tbsp honey
1 tbsp soy sauce
juice of 1 lime
1 tbsp coconut oil
1 red pepper, finely sliced
½ courgette, diced
a handful of broccoli, broken into small florets
a handful of chopped scallions
300g straight-to-wok rice noodles

The honey and soy sauce in this recipe make a delicious glaze that really locks in the flavour of the salmon. This recipe makes good use of your time too: while the salmon roasts in the oven, you cook the stir-fry and noodles. It's a delicious and nutritious dinner – fast!

Preheat the oven to 180°C/350°F/gas 4. Place the salmon fillets skin-side down on a non-stick ovenproof dish. Smear the butter over the salmon fillets. Mix the honey, soy sauce and lime juice in a small bowl. Pour half of this dressing over the salmon fillets. Place the salmon fillets in the oven and roast them for 15 minutes or until cooked through.

Meanwhile, melt the coconut oil in a large pan over a medium-high heat. Add all of the vegetables and stir-fry for about 5 minutes. Add the noodles and the remaining dressing. Stir well and cook for 3 minutes or until the noodles are heated through.

Divide the stir-fry between warmed serving bowls. Top with the roasted salmon and serve.

PROTEIN 33G	
FAT (SATURATED) 33G (17.8G)	
CARB 126G	
FIBRE 4.3G	
CAL 941	

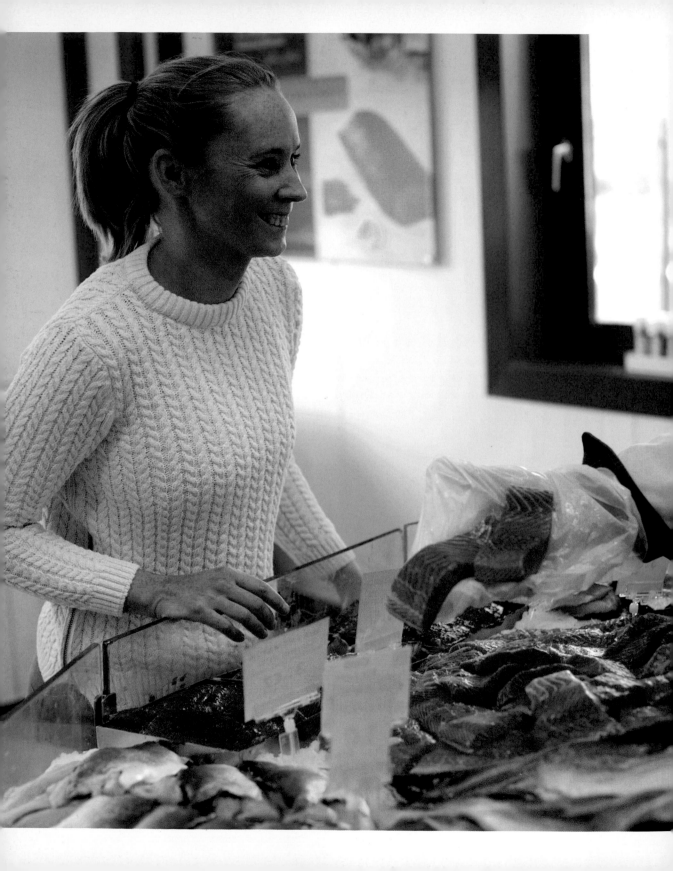

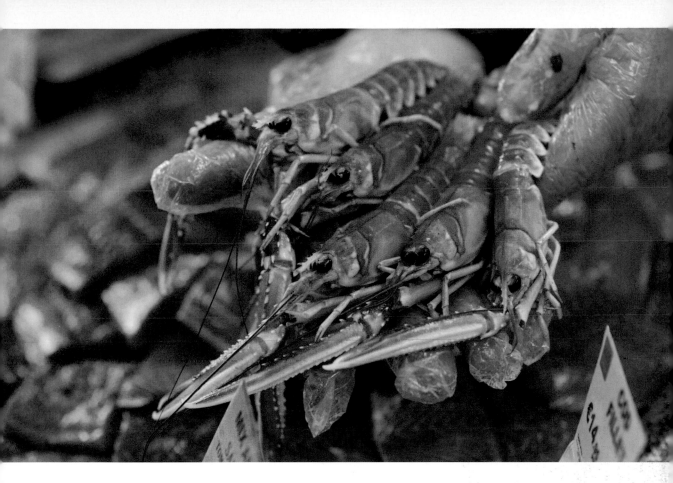

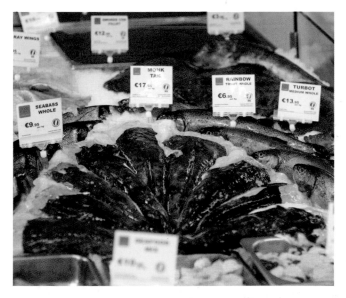

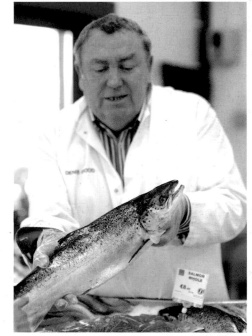

EASY-PEASY SALMON BAKE

**PREP TIME: 5 MIN
COOK TIME:
   15-20 MIN**

olive oil
1 carrot, peeled and
   finely sliced
1 onion, sliced
1 red pepper, sliced
1 yellow pepper, sliced
½ courgette, diced
4 garlic cloves, crushed
4 tbsp chopped chives
4 lemon slices
4 × 100g salmon fillets,
   skinned
salt and pepper
4 medium-sized baked
   sweet potatoes, to serve
4 tbsp natural yoghurt,
   to serve

When I'm not sure what to have for dinner, I often end up baking some fish – and my recipe will be some variation on this one. It's quick and the ingredients are fairly interchangeable: cod and hake are just as delicious as salmon. I serve the fish with a baked sweet potato and a dollop of natural yoghurt. It is one easy-peasy satisfying meal!

Preheat the oven to 180°C/350°F/gas 4. Lightly oil a large ovenproof dish. Place the vegetables and chives in the dish and arrange the lemon slices on top. Lay the salmon fillets on top of the lemon slices. Drizzle over one tablespoon of olive oil and season well. Cover the dish with foil and place it in the oven for 15–20 minutes, or until the salmon is cooked through. Divide the salmon and vegetables between warmed serving plates. Serve with baked sweet potatoes and natural yoghurt.

PROTEIN 29G

FAT (SATURATED) 21G (4.1G)

CARB 52G

FIBRE 6.7G

CAL 528

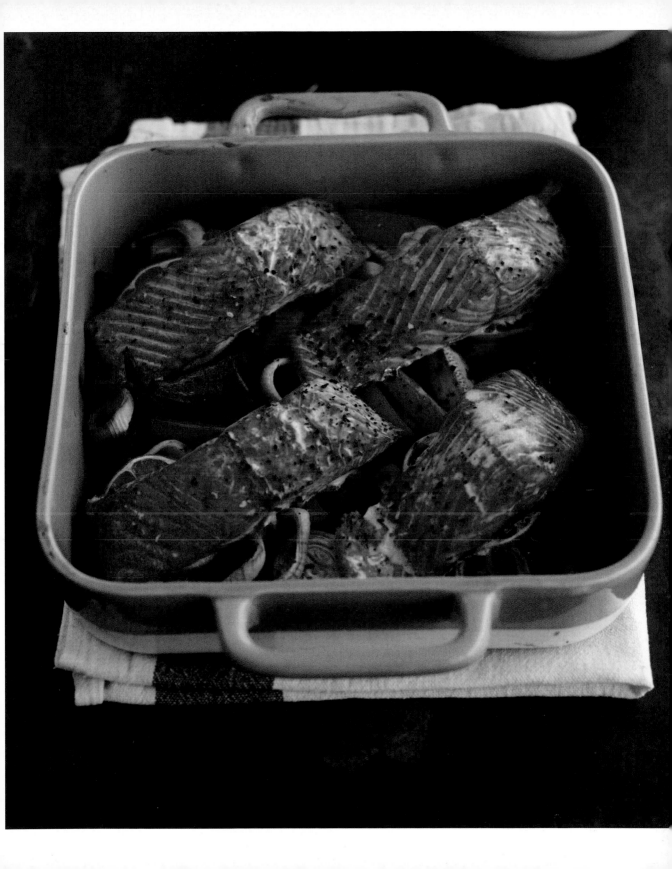

MEDITERRANEAN SALMON & SPAGHETTI

PREP TIME: 5 MIN
COOK TIME:
15-20 MIN

4 × 100g salmon fillets,
  skinned
2 tbsp butter
salt and pepper
200g wholewheat
  spaghetti
2 tbsp olive oil
5 garlic cloves, crushed
12 cherry tomatoes,
  halved
2 tbsp capers, rinsed and
  roughly chopped
2 tbsp grated Parmesan
a handful of basil leaves
2 handfuls of rocket
  leaves

This is a super-quick supper that's full of Mediterranean flavour. While the spaghetti is hearty and filling, the sauce is refreshing and light. This recipe is not suitable for the freezer but the leftovers are great the next day as a cold pasta salad, which is a handy option if you're dining *al desko* or want a hassle-free lunch at home. If you want, you can double the quantity of salmon and bake in bulk: leftover roasted salmon is a fantastic and nutritious sandwich-filler.

Preheat the oven to 180°C/350°F/gas 4. Place the salmon fillets, skin-side down, in an ovenproof dish. Rub the butter over the salmon fillets and season well. Cover the dish with foil and place it in the oven for 15 minutes or until the salmon is cooked through.

Meanwhile, cook the spaghetti according to the instructions on the package.

Heat the oil in a large pan over a low heat. Add the garlic and cook for 2 minutes. Stir in the tomatoes, capers and Parmesan. Tear the basil leaves and stir them into the pan. Toss in the cooked pasta and mix well. Divide the pasta between warmed serving bowls and top with the cooked salmon. Divide the rocket evenly between the bowls and serve.

PROTEIN 29G

FAT (SATURATED) 46G (11G)

CARB 12.9G

FIBRE 2.7G

CAL 590

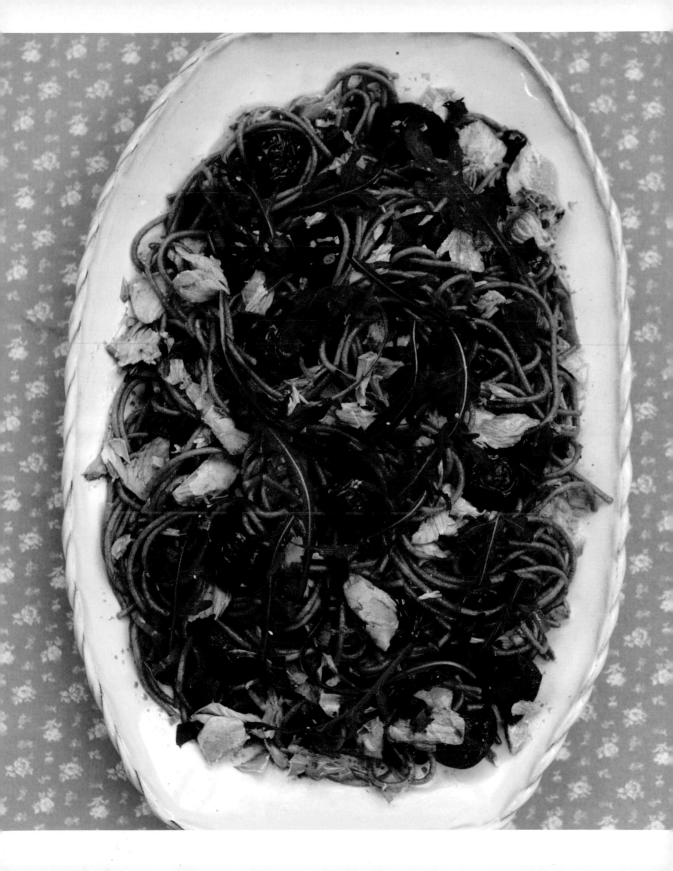

FIT FOODIE NUT ROAST

PREP TIME: 10 MIN
COOK TIME: 50 MIN

100g almonds, flaked
100g cashews
50g pine nuts
75g Cheddar, grated
70g dried apricots,
   roughly chopped
2 eggs, lightly beaten
1 tbsp olive oil
3 leeks, trimmed and
   finely sliced
1 onion, finely chopped
1 medium potato, peeled
   and grated
1 tbsp chopped rosemary

I used to think that nut roast was a dish reserved for vegetarians – not for meat-lovers like me. But I changed my mind after eating a delicious nut roast in a vegetarian restaurant. Coming up with my own version took a few attempts but now I'm very proud of this recipe. Fit Foodie Nut Roast combines two of my major food heroes: nuts and eggs. It's equally delicious served cold or hot and makes a great dinner and a gorgeous lunch the next day too. In summer, it goes really well with a green salad and a nice chutney; in winter, it's delicious with roasted vegetables on the side.

Preheat the oven to 180°C/350°F/gas 4. You will need a 900g (2lb) silicone loaf pan. Blitz the nuts in a food processor until they look like rough breadcrumbs. Tip the nuts into a large mixing bowl. Add the Cheddar, apricots and eggs and stir to combine.

Heat the oil in a large pan over a medium heat. Add the leeks, onion, potato and rosemary and cook for about 10 minutes, stirring frequently. Tip the cooked vegetables into the bowl with the nut mixture. Stir well to combine. Scrape the mixture into the loaf pan. Bake for about 30 minutes, until the loaf is firm when pressed gently.

Remove the Nut Roast from the oven and leave to cool in the loaf pan for 10 minutes. Carefully remove the Nut Roast from the loaf pan. Slice and serve.

PROTEIN 22G

FAT (SATURATED) 45G (11.1G)

CARB 26G

FIBRE 9.1G

CAL 617

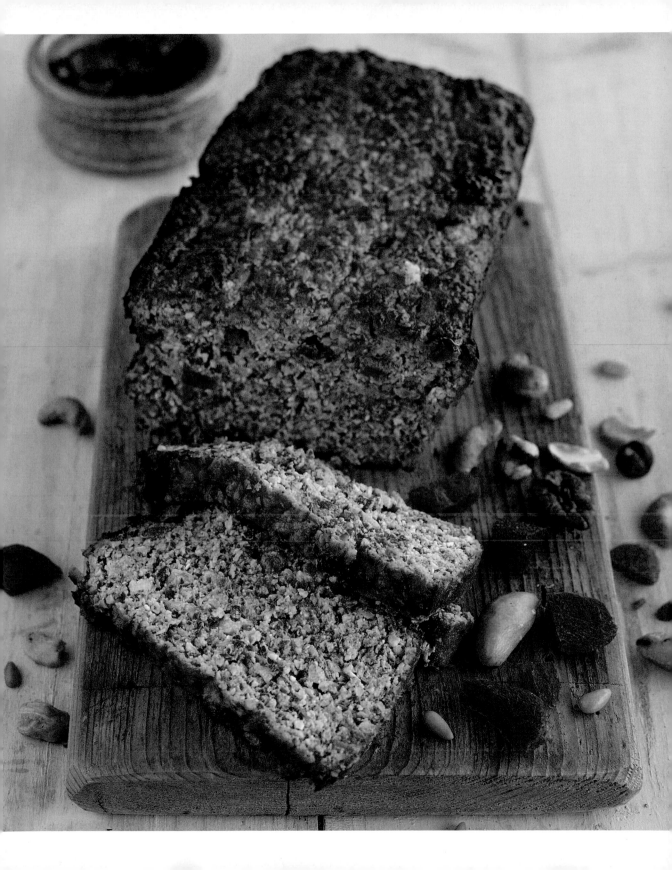

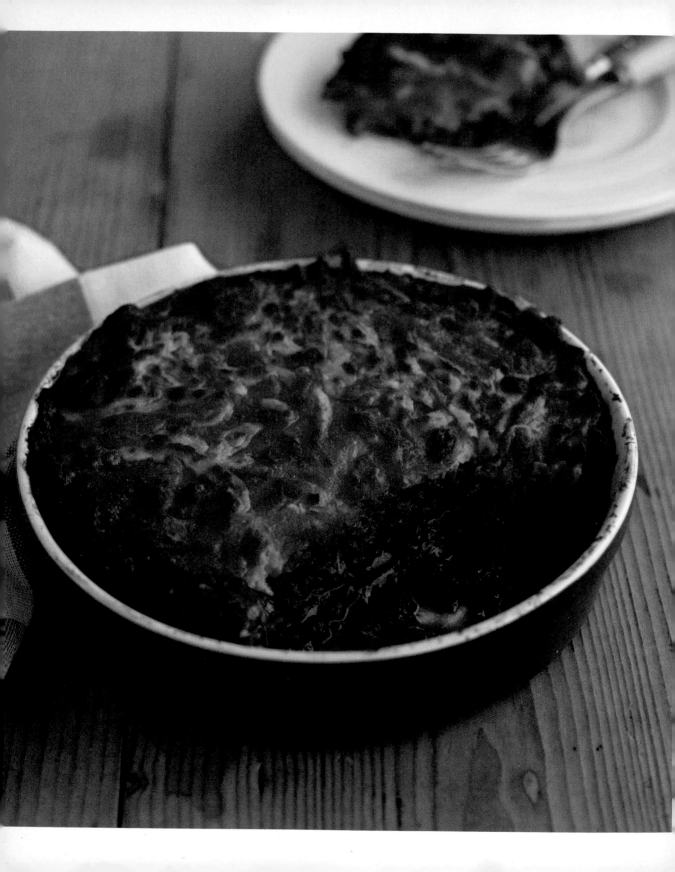

TOMATO & AUBERGINE BAKE

PREP TIME: 10 MIN
COOK TIME: 35 MIN

2 aubergines, cut
   lengthways into thin
   slices
olive oil
salt and pepper
2 onions, finely chopped
5 garlic cloves, crushed
400g tin of chopped
   tomatoes
2 tbsp tomato purée
a handful of basil leaves,
   torn
3 eggs, beaten
30g mozzarella, sliced
1 tbsp grated Parmesan

This dish gives you so many options for dinner. It's delicious by itself or served alongside some chicken, fish or couscous. If you want a freezer-friendly version, just leave out the egg topping but cook everything else as normal. Sometimes I make this bake without the egg and say that I'm going to freeze it. But then I end up reheating it for dinner for three days straight and it never makes it to the freezer because it's just too good . . .

Preheat the oven to 160°C/325°F/gas 3. Lightly brush both sides of the aubergine slices with olive oil and season well. Divide the aubergine slices between two baking trays and bake for 12 minutes, turning once during cooking.

Meanwhile, heat a tablespoon of olive oil in a large pan on a medium heat. Add the onions and cook for 5 minutes. Add the garlic and cook for 2 minutes. Stir in the tomatoes and tomato purée. Remove the aubergine slices from the oven and increase the heat to 180°C/350°F/gas 4.

Layer half of the aubergine slices in the bottom of a large ovenproof dish. Add the basil to the tomato sauce and stir well. Pour the sauce over the aubergines in the dish. Add the remaining aubergine slices in an even layer. Pour the beaten eggs on top and scatter over the mozzarella and Parmesan. Bake for 15–20 minutes. Divide the bake between warmed serving bowls.

PROTEIN 8.6G	
FAT (SATURATED) 21G (8.4G)	
CARB 14.3G	
FIBRE 2.8G	
CAL 331	

BUTTERNUT & BEAN STEW

PREP TIME: 10 MIN
COOK TIME: 30 MIN

1 tbsp coconut oil
4 garlic cloves, crushed
1 onion, finely chopped
½ chilli, finely chopped
a thumb-sized piece of
   fresh ginger, grated
2 cardamom pods, whole
1 tbsp cumin seeds
1 tbsp turmeric
1 star anise
1 butternut squash,
   peeled, deseeded, diced
1 aubergine, diced
400g tin of chopped
   tomatoes
2 tbsp soy sauce
1 tbsp honey
400g tin of mixed beans
a handful of coriander
   leaves
4 tbsp flaked almonds
4 tbsp Greek yoghurt

This vegetable stew is full of delicious flavours and textures. The beans provide lots of protein and vitamin B and make this a hearty and nourishing meal. It's a one-pot dish, so you won't have to face a lot of washing-up after dinner (always a plus). If you wanted to make this stew even more substantial, you could serve it with rice or couscous. It's one of those dishes that tastes even better on the second day: the leftovers are fantastic.

Melt the coconut oil in a large pan over a medium heat. Add the garlic, onion, chilli and ginger and cook for about 5 minutes. Stir frequently and add a splash of water if the pan gets dry. Stir in the spices and cook for 2 minutes. Add the butternut and aubergine and cook for 2 minutes, stirring frequently. Add the tomatoes, soy sauce and honey and stir well. Cover the pan and simmer for about 30 minutes, stirring occasionally.

When the vegetables are tender, stir in the beans and heat through. Divide the stew between warmed serving bowls. Sprinkle over the coriander and flaked almonds. Top with a dollop of Greek yoghurt and serve.

PROTEIN 16.7G	
FAT (SATURATED) 19.6G (9.6G)	
CARB 46G	
FIBRE 10.9G	
CAL 454	

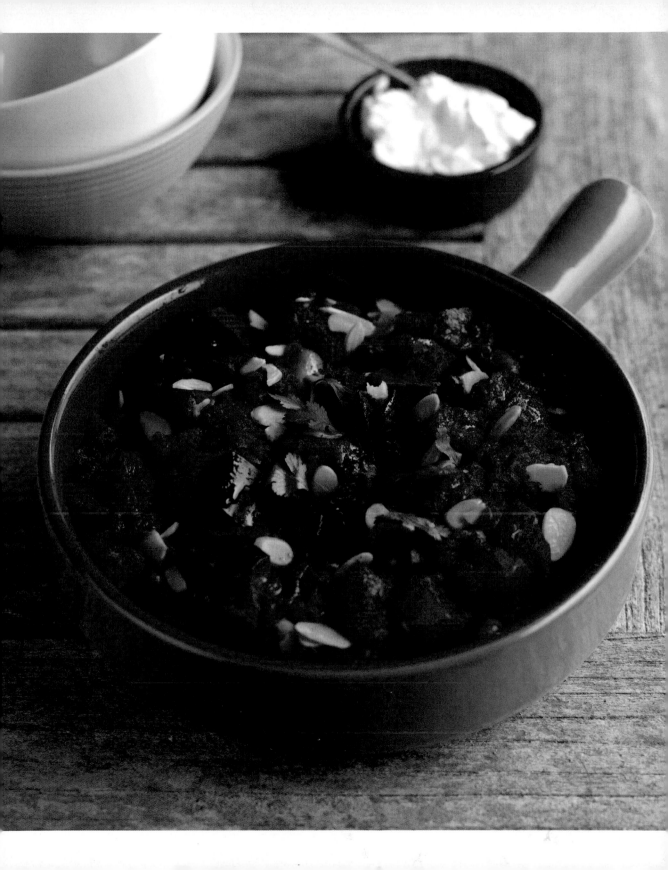

MAKING FRIENDS WITH YOUR FREEZER

I consider freezer-stocking to be an important survival skill. The freezer can be a fantastic source of healthy midweek dinners and if you have a well-stocked one, you can eat well no matter how busy things get. It's a great feeling to come home after a busy day to find a delicious dinner defrosted in the fridge and ready to be transformed into a hot meal in minutes. If you don't have a freezer, consider investing in one – even a small one. If you do have a freezer, make the most of it. Here are my tips for becoming firm friends with your freezer.

FREEZER BASICS

GETTING IT IN

As soon as your big batch of freshly cooked dinner has cooled, pop the leftovers into a freezer-safe container. Make sure that you have labels so that you can write the name of the dish and the date it was cooked. There are few things more frustrating than a freezer full of mystery foods.

GETTING IT OUT

It's great to start the working day by going to your freezer and choosing a delicious dish to defrost for dinner. The only challenge is remembering to defrost it in the first place. So set a reminder on your phone or write a sticky note for yourself: do whatever you need to do to get that dinner defrosting on time!

GETTING IT RIGHT

Remember food safety tips when using your freezer. Don't leave food in your freezer for too long: I try to use up everything within 3 months. Defrost food in the fridge (not on the counter). Never re-freeze defrosted food. And if you have a power cut, keep that freezer door closed! The food should hold for a day or so.

KEEPING IT CLUTTER-FREE

Once you start using your freezer regularly, you'll come to really rely on it: so you'll need to keep it clutter-free. Organize your freezer into sections, such as meat, fish, vegetables, fruit and complete meals. Then you'll always be ready to grab something and go!

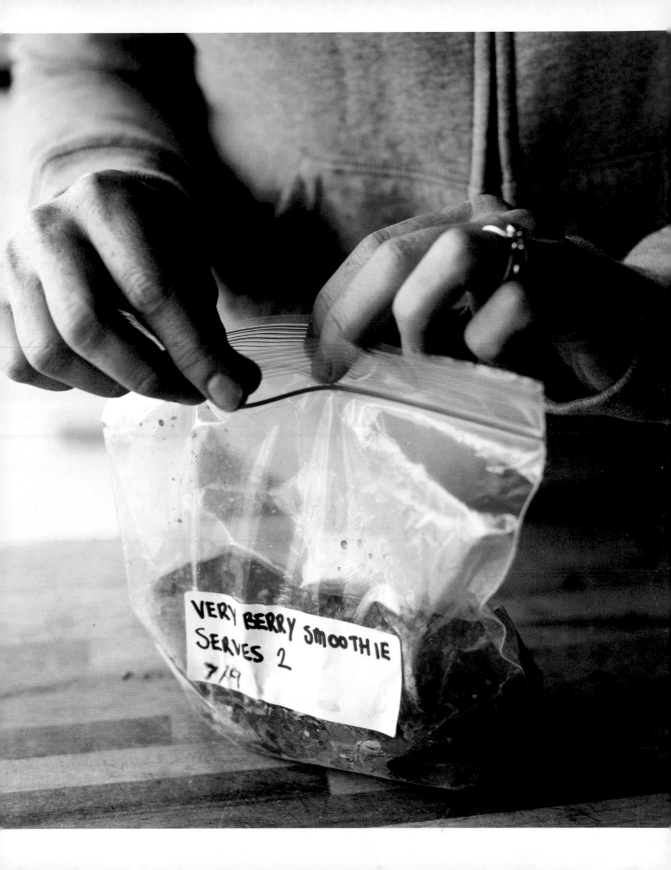

FREEZER FOODS

VEGETABLES

Some people assume that frozen vegetables are inferior to fresh vegetables, but it's just not true. Vegetables that are frozen from fresh retain a huge amount of their nutritional value. And having a freezer full of prepped vegetables is a major step towards having a healthier lifestyle. There's no compromise on taste either: frozen vegetables are full of flavour and can brighten up any dinnertime.

FRUIT

Most fruits do really well in the freezer, especially if you want to use them in smoothies. If you're feeling super-organized, you can chop up the fruit for a particular smoothie, put it in a ziplock bag, write the name of the smoothie on the bag and throw it in the freezer. You'll have cool, fresh smoothies on tap.

GINGER

Fresh ginger never has to go to waste. Buy it in bulk, peel it and grate it. Then, taking one teaspoon at a time, scoop the grated ginger onto a baking sheet lined with parchment paper. Freeze until solid. Stack the frozen ginger pieces in an airtight container and store in the freezer. You will have ginger bombs ready to throw straight from the freezer into your cooking pot!

GARLIC

You never want to be without garlic. Fortunately, it freezes really well. Crush or finely chop several bulbs of garlic. Then tip the whole lot into a ziplock bag. You'll have a big ball of garlic in your freezer, ready for you to break off pieces as you need them.

CHILLIES & HERBS

Chillies can bring something special to a meal, so it's a good idea to have chopped chillies ready to go. Deseed and finely chop several chillies. Spoon the chopped chillies into an ice-cube tray, leaving enough room to top each cube with water. Freeze until solid. Whenever your recipe calls for chopped chilli, just drop a frozen chilli cube straight into the cooking pot. This trick also works with fresh herbs.

STOCK

If you're going to make stock (see p. 205), make the biggest batch your kitchen can handle: you'll always find use for good stock! Freeze the stock in smaller portions so that you can use what you need when you need it.

BREAD

Bread freezes really well. If you bake Almond, Pine Nut & Hazelnut Bread (see p. 154), slice the loaf and freeze the slices. You can take a slice straight from the freezer and pop it in the toaster. Delicious, healthy toast in minutes! Keep a packet of wholemeal pittas in the freezer too.

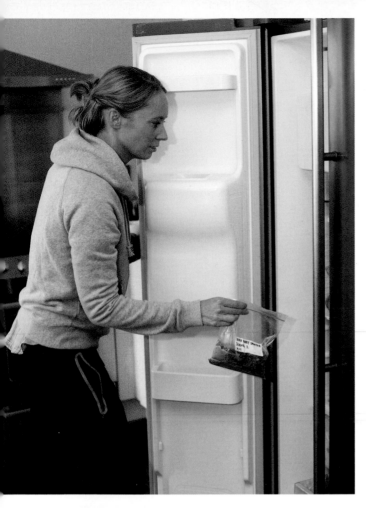

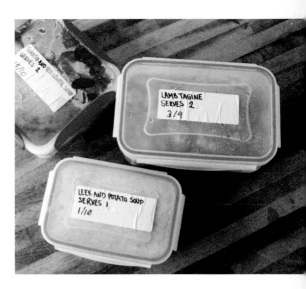

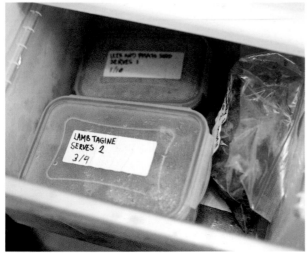

MEAT

We all have busy lives, so it's unlikely we can go to the butcher every time we want to buy fresh meat for a recipe. This is where the freezer comes into its own. Fill your freezer with a variety of cuts of meat: you won't be stuck for ideas at dinnertime.

FISH

Fresh fish is delicious: enjoy it whenever you get the chance. But remember that fish freezes really well too. Keep your freezer stocked with fish. I always have plenty of oily fish in my freezer: it's like omega-3 goodness on ice.

'READY MEALS'

So many Fit Foodie recipes are dinners that freeze well. Look for this symbol throughout the book: ❄. Make sure that you have a selection of these meals in your freezer so that you're ready for those days when only a 'ready meal' will do!

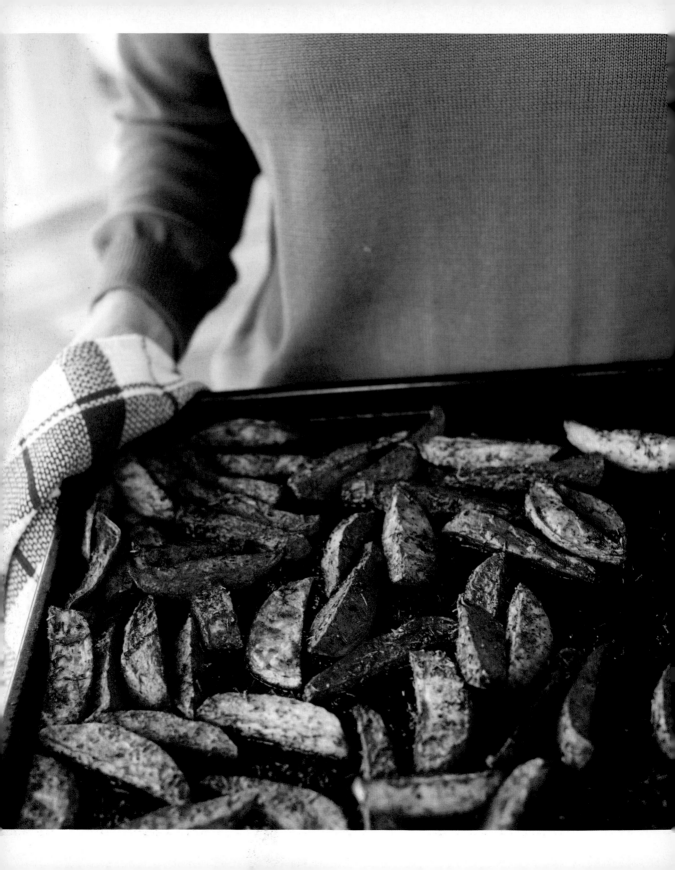

SIDES & SNACKS

MINTY PEAS

BAKE-N-SMASH MASH

HERBED POTATO WEDGES

SURPLUS SPUDS SALAD

ROASTED PEPPERS

SALSA VERDE

HUMMUS WITH A KICK

MANGO SALSAS

MINTY PEAS

PREP TIME: 2 MIN
COOK TIME: 5 MIN

3 tbsp butter
150g frozen baby peas
a handful of mint leaves,
  chopped

When I'm out to dinner, I'll often order a side of peas – just to see how the chef has spruced things up. This is my idea for livening up your peas and making them a side dish to look forward to. In terms of their nutritional benefits, peas don't get the credit they deserve. They are small but mighty: packed full of protein, antioxidants and fibre. The humble pea is well deserving of a place on your plate!

Melt the butter in a large pot over a medium heat. Add the frozen peas, mint and a tablespoon of water. Simmer for about 5 minutes, until the peas are heated through, and serve.

PROTEIN 4.8G

FAT (SATURATED) 12.9G (7.9G)

CARB 7G

FIBRE 5.5G

CAL 176

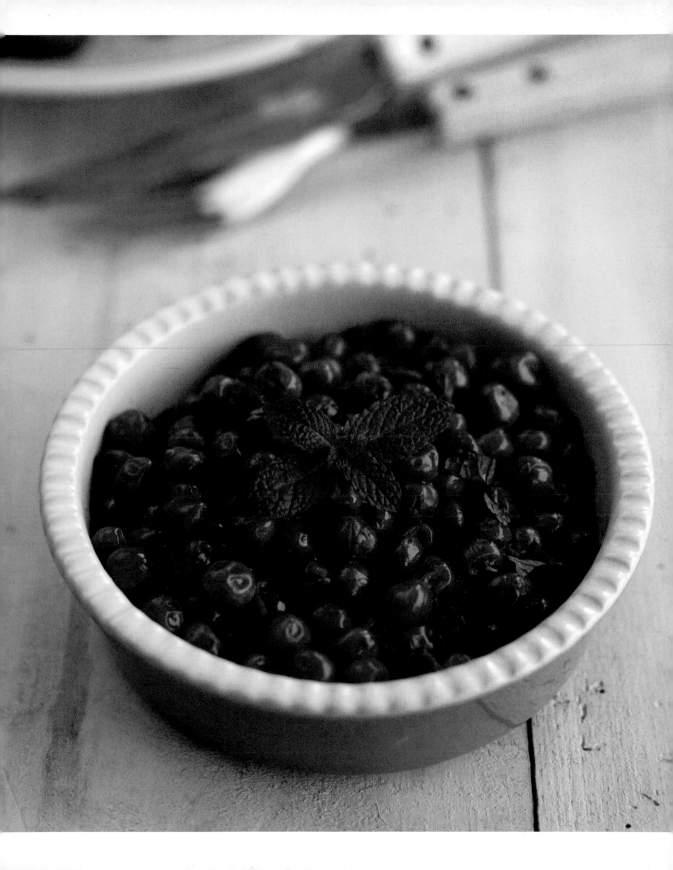

BAKE-N-SMASH MASH

I'm always trying to find ways to make the most out of the time I spend in the kitchen – that's how these Bake-n-Smash Mash recipes came about. Whenever you find yourself using the oven, check to see if there's room to bake some potatoes at the same time. You'll need about 45 minutes for the Sweet Potato Mash and about 75 minutes for the Regular Mash. So don't leave a stew sitting all alone in the oven: throw in a potato to keep it company! It makes good sense to use your oven for two things at once. And if you don't want to eat the mash straight away, store it in an airtight container in the fridge for a few days. Both of these recipes reheat well and keep the beautiful texture of freshly cooked mash. These recipes really are the ultimate in low-maintenance mash.

SWEET POTATO MASH

PREP TIME: 5 MIN
COOK TIME: 45 MIN

1 small sweet potato, washed, dried and pricked all over with a fork
1 tsp maple syrup
½ tsp fresh thyme leaves
salt and pepper

Preheat the oven to 180°C/350°F/gas 4. Wrap the sweet potato loosely in foil and place it on a baking tray. Bake for 45 minutes or until the sweet potato is tender when pricked with a fork. Remove the sweet potato from the oven, remove the foil, and place the sweet potato on a wire rack to cool slightly. Peel the sweet potato and place the flesh in a large bowl. Mash well and stir in the maple syrup and thyme. Season to taste and serve.

PROTEIN 1.8G
FAT (SATURATED) 0.6G (0.2G)
CARB 41G
FIBRE 3G
CAL 183

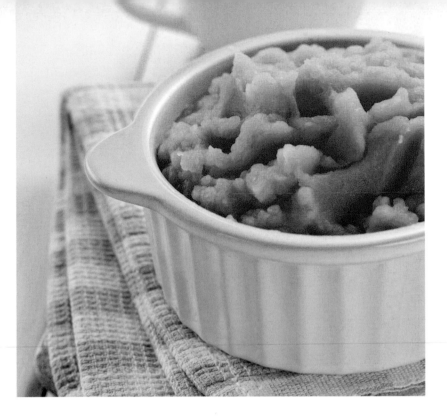

PREP TIME: 5 MIN
COOK TIME:
  1 HR 15 MIN

1 medium baking potato,
  washed, dried and
  pricked all over with
  a fork
1 tsp butter
1 tsp warm milk
1 tsp chopped chives
salt and pepper

REGULAR MASH

Preheat the oven to 180°C/350°F/gas 4. Wrap the potato loosely in foil and place it on a baking tray. Bake for 75 minutes or until the potato is tender when pricked with a fork. Remove the potato from the oven, remove the foil, and place the potato on a wire rack to cool slightly. Peel the potato and place the flesh in a large bowl. Mash well and stir in the butter, milk and chives. Season to taste and serve.

PROTEIN 4.8G	
FAT (SATURATED) 4.7G (2.9G)	
CARB 35G	
FIBRE 4.4G	
CAL 214	

HERBED POTATO WEDGES

Potato wedges make such a versatile side dish – they're delicious with meat, fish or vegetables. These wedges are great to make pre- or post-workout, if you want to steer clear of junk food and still get a savoury hit.

PREP TIME: 5 MIN
COOK TIME: 40 MIN

4 medium-sized potatoes, scrubbed (not peeled) and cut into wedges
2 tbsp olive oil
4 tbsp dried herbs (oregano, basil, tarragon and sage work well)
salt and pepper

REGULAR WEDGES

Preheat the oven to 200°C/400°F/gas 6. You will need two large baking trays.

Place the potato wedges, oil and herbs in a large mixing bowl. Use your hands to give each potato wedge a coating of oil and herbs. Spread the potato wedges on the baking trays and roast for about 40 minutes, turning once. Divide the potato wedges between serving bowls and season to taste.

PREP TIME: 5 MIN
COOK TIME: 40 MIN

4 medium-sized sweet potatoes, scrubbed (not peeled) and cut into wedges
2 tbsp olive oil
4 tbsp dried herbs (oregano, basil, tarragon and sage work well)
salt and pepper

SWEET POTATO WEDGES

Preheat the oven to 200°C/400°F/gas 6. You will need two large baking trays.

Place the sweet potato wedges, oil and herbs in a large mixing bowl. Use your hands to give each sweet potato wedge a coating of oil and herbs. Spread the sweet potato wedges on the baking trays and roast for about 30 minutes, turning once. Divide the sweet potato wedges between serving bowls and season to taste.

REGULAR WEDGES	SWEET WEDGES
PROTEIN 1.3G	PROTEIN 1.7G
FAT (SATURATED) 13G (1.9G)	FAT (SATURATED) 13.1G (2G)
CARB 12.4G	CARB 27G
FIBRE 1.4G	FIBRE 3.1G
CAL 176	CAL 239

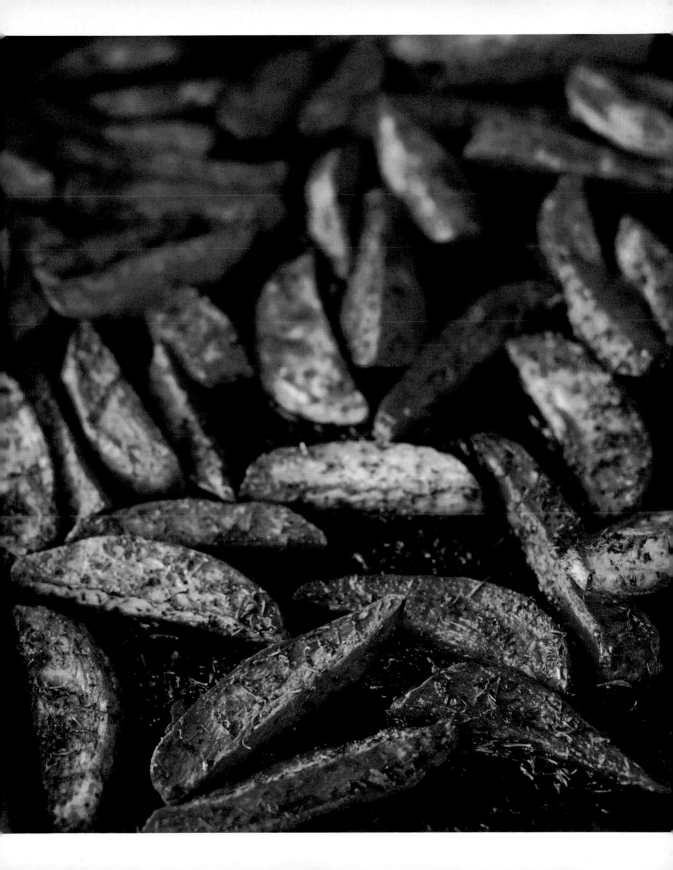

SURPLUS SPUDS SALAD

PREP TIME: 3 MIN
COOK TIME: 5 MIN

5 medium-sized new
  potatoes, scrubbed,
  boiled or steamed until
  tender, cooled
1 apple, peeled, cored
  and finely chopped
50g walnuts, chopped
250g natural yoghurt
juice of ½ lime
a handful of mint leaves,
  chopped

If you're going to cook potatoes, I think it's worth your while cooking a few extra because you can always use the leftovers as a base for another meal. This Surplus Spuds Salad is a great way to use up leftover potatoes. Serve this side salad with chicken or fish and you've got a fast and delicious meal with very little hassle. This salad keeps fresh for a day or two in an airtight container in the fridge.

Use a potato masher or fork to roughly crush the potatoes in a large bowl. Mix the apple, walnuts, yoghurt, lime and mint in a medium bowl. Add the yoghurt mixture to the potatoes and mix well. Scrape the potato salad into a serving bowl and enjoy.

PROTEIN 15.5G

FAT (SATURATED) 22G (2.7G)

CARB 36G

FIBRE 4.9G

CAL 421

ROASTED PEPPERS

**COOK TIME: 1 HR
(INCLUDES COOLING)**

4 red or yellow peppers,
  whole
2 tbsp olive oil
1 tbsp fresh herbs,
  chopped (rosemary
  and thyme work well)

This recipe is based on an Ina Garten method that works a treat. It's the easiest possible way to roast peppers: you just put the peppers on an ovenproof dish and roast them. As soon as the peppers come out of the oven, you cover the dish tightly with tin foil and leave it to sit. This creates a steam that makes the peppers easy to peel and deseed. Roasted peppers are a great fridge-filler. They can be used to make hummus, and they're delicious in salads and sandwiches too. Coated with a little olive oil, the roasted peppers keep for up to two weeks.

Preheat the oven to 230°C/450°F/gas 8. Lay the peppers on their sides in an ovenproof dish. Cook the peppers for 15 minutes. Turn the peppers and cook them for 15–20 minutes more. The peppers are ready when they are completely wrinkled, charred and soft.

Remove the peppers from the oven and immediately cover the dish with tin foil. Seal the tin foil tightly around the edges so that no steam can escape. Set aside for 30 minutes.

Remove the stem, skins and seeds from each pepper. Place the roasted peppers in an airtight container, stir in the herbs and drizzle over the olive oil. Store in the fridge for up to two weeks.

PROTEIN 1.6G

FAT (SATURATED) 6.9G (1.1G)

CARB 9.9G

FIBRE 3G

CAL 116

SALSA VERDE

PREP TIME: 10 MIN

10 Brazil nuts (pine nuts
   and cashew nuts also
   work well)
4 garlic cloves, crushed
1 tbsp capers
a handful of mint leaves
a handful of parsley
a handful of basil leaves
4 tbsp olive oil
1 tbsp red wine vinegar
3 tsp Dijon mustard
salt and pepper

Salsa verde is the perfect summer sauce. It's bursting with flavour and it goes with just about everything: chicken, fish and any vegetable. Some people insist that you have to make this by hand; others insist that it should be done with a mortar and pestle. I just throw everything into a food processor and it works beautifully. Store your salsa verde in the fridge, where it will keep for several days in an airtight container.

Place the Brazil nuts in a bowl of warm water to soften for about 10 minutes. Drain the Brazil nuts and place them in a food processor along with the remaining ingredients. Blitz for about 30 seconds, until the salsa verde is smooth.

PROTEIN 9.5G	
FAT (SATURATED) 84G (9.3G)	
CARB 5.9G	
FIBRE 2.4G	
CAL 826	

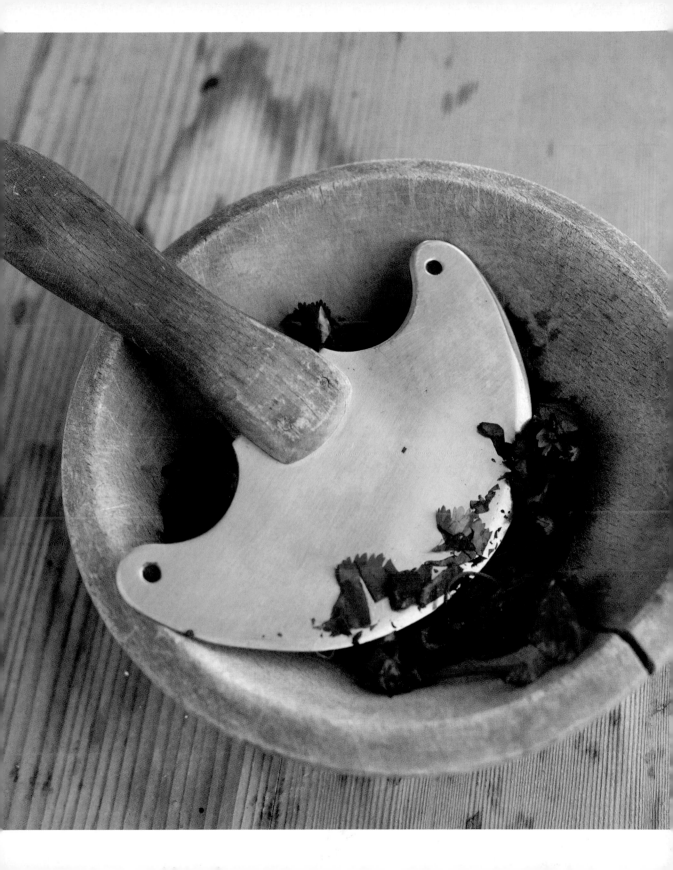

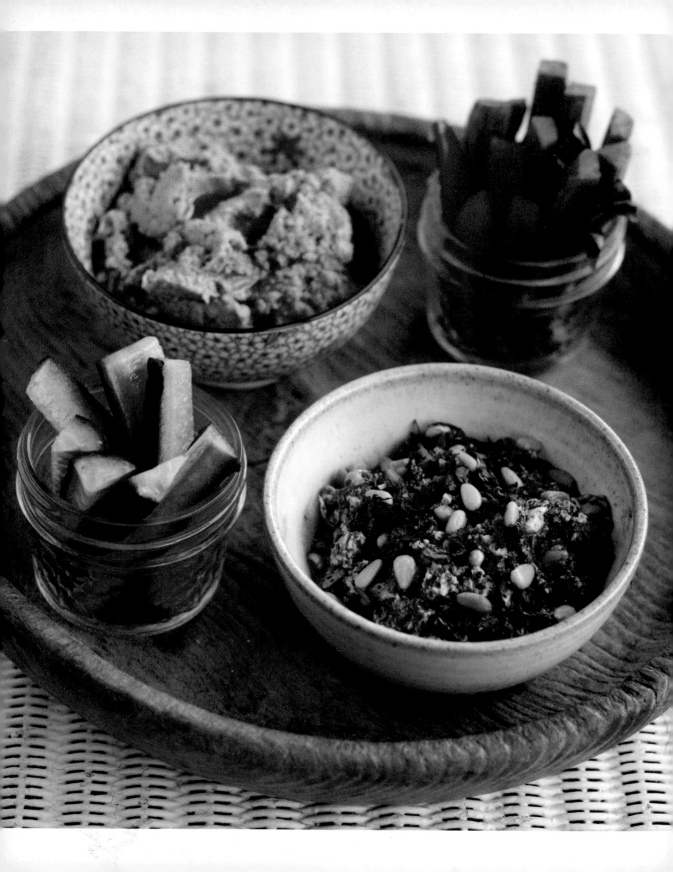

HUMMUS WITH A KICK

PREP TIME: 10 MIN

400g tin of chickpeas,
   drained and rinsed
4 large garlic cloves,
   finely grated
zest and juice of 1 lemon
4 tbsp olive oil
1–2 tsp honey
1–2 tsp tahini
1–2 tsp Tabasco sauce
salt and black pepper

This is hummus with a real kick! If you don't like it too spicy, you could always tone down the garlic and Tabasco. This hummus goes really well with cucumber, celery, peppers and carrot sticks. It's the thing I reach for when I'm hungry and I need something quick and tasty, but I don't want to spoil my dinner. You can freeze hummus. I've never tried with this one – but that's because I always manage to get through the leftovers within a day or two. Of course, if I serve this to friends or family – even if I make a double batch – there's not a hope of leftovers!

Place all of the ingredients in a food processer and blitz until you have a smooth hummus. If you like a thin consistency, add another teaspoon of olive oil or water. Scrape the hummus into serving bowls and brace yourself.

PROTEIN 7.9G	
FAT (SATURATED) 16.9G (2.3G)	
CARB 17.2G	
FIBRE 5.2G	
CAL 265	

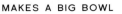

MANGO SALSAS

These mango salsas add flavour, colour and a nutritional boost to so many dishes! The first salsa is cool and refreshing, while the second one is hot and zingy. They will liven up a sandwich at lunchtime and will also taste great on grilled chicken or fish. Both of these salsas can be made in minutes.

THE COOL ONE

PREP TIME: 5 MIN

1 mango, peeled and
  diced
½ cucumber, peeled,
  deseeded and diced
a handful of mint leaves,
  chopped
juice of ½ lime
1 tsp apple cider vinegar

Place all of the ingredients in a medium bowl. Toss well to combine. Transfer the salsa to a serving bowl.

THE HOT ONE

PREP TIME: 5 MIN

1 mango, peeled and
  diced
1 chilli, deseeded and
  finely chopped
a handful of coriander
  leaves, chopped
a handful of mint leaves,
  chopped
a handful of finely
  chopped scallions
juice of 1 lime

Place all of the ingredients in a medium bowl. Toss well to combine. Transfer the salsa to a serving bowl.

THE COOL ONE	THE HOT ONE
PROTEIN 4.1G	PROTEIN 2.8G
FAT (SATURATED) 0.8G (0.2G)	FAT (SATURATED) 0.7G (0.2G)
CARB 37G	CARB 34G
FIBRE 8.8G	FIBRE 7.3G
CAL 191	CAL 170

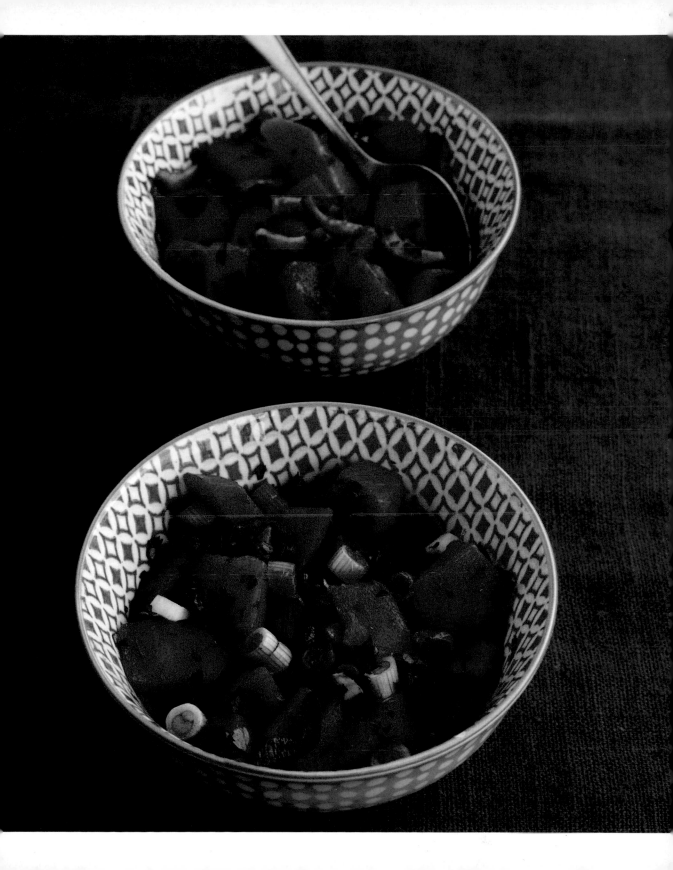

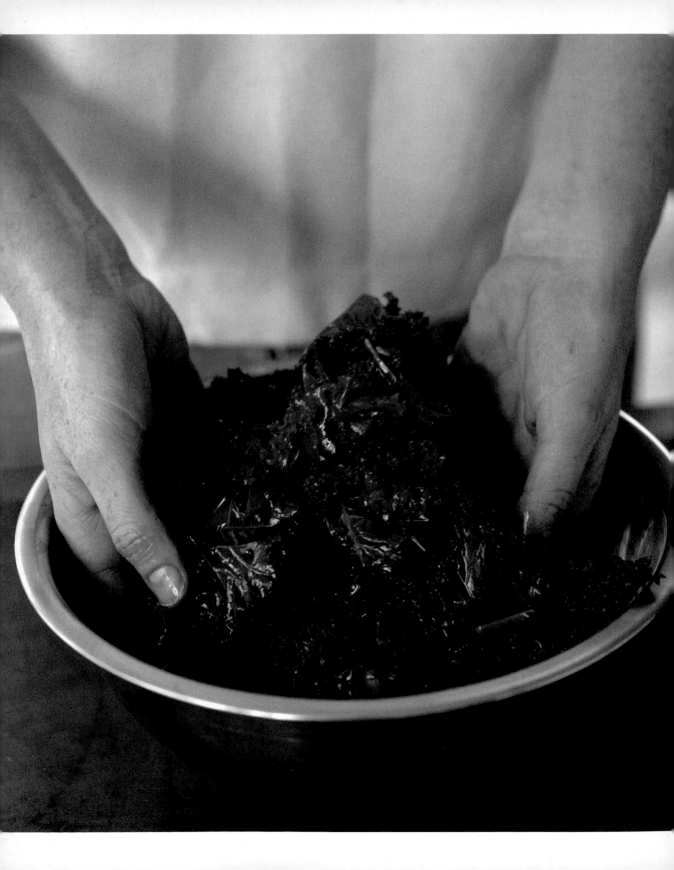

SUPER SNACKS

KALE KRISPS

APPLE & CHEDDER STACKS

PECAN & DATE LOAF

ALMOND, PINE NUT & HAZELNUT BREAD

NUTTY BANANA BREAD

BOOSTER BARS

COCOA & HAZELNUT BOMBS

CHOCOLATE & COCOUNT ENERGY BARS

ORANGE & DATE ENERGY BALLS

BANANA SQUARES

POSH NUTS

KALE KRISPS

PREP TIME: 10 MIN
COOK TIME: 10 MIN

200g kale, tough stalks
    removed (200g is the
    weight without stalks)
4 tbsp olive oil
1 tsp chilli flakes (1 tbsp
    if you want a real kick)
salt and pepper

I used to be a kale-crisp hater. My logic was this: if I want to eat a bag of crisps, I'll just buy a bag of crisps. But then I saw kale crisps everywhere and, rather than spend a fortune on a small bag, I figured I'd have a go at making them myself. They are actually really tasty – surprisingly tasty. Now I'm a kale-crisp lover. Could you be one too?

Preheat the oven to 200°C/400°F/gas 6.

Wash the kale and dry it thoroughly. Tear larger leaves into crisp-sized pieces. Place the kale in a large mixing bowl. Pour in the oil and toss well. Add the chilli flakes and seasoning and mix well. Spread the kale on a large silicone baking sheet. Bake for 10 minutes or until the crisps become crispy!

Remove the crisps from the oven and allow them to cool slightly on the tray. Season to taste and serve.

PROTEIN 3.6G	
FAT (SATURATED) 27G (3.8G)	
CARB 2.3G	
FIBRE 4.1G	
CAL 274	

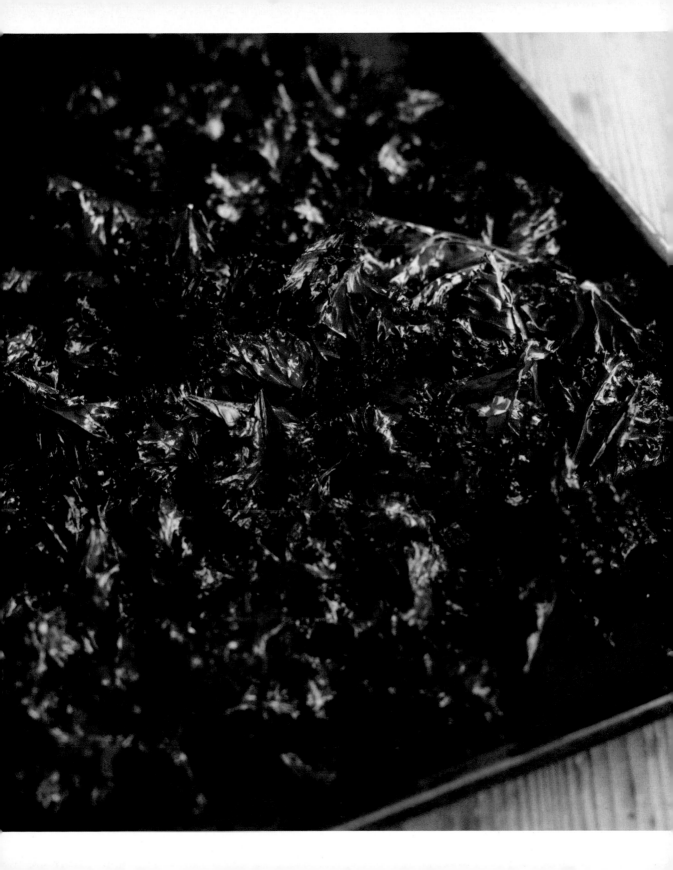

APPLE & CHEDDAR STACKS

PREP TIME: 2 MIN

2 oat cakes
25g white Cheddar, finely
   sliced
½ apple, finely sliced

Even if supplies run really low in my house, I'll usually have the three ingredients needed for this quick snack. I turn to these Apple & Cheddar Stacks when I'm feeling peckish and I need something to tide me over until I can make my next meal. The combination of apple and Cheddar really hits the spot – and the oat cakes will keep hunger at bay until you can rustle up something more substantial.

Place the oat cakes on a small plate. Layer alternate slices of Cheddar and apple on each oat cake until all of the ingredients are used up – then serve.

PROTEIN 8.6G	
FAT (SATURATED) 11.6G (6G)	
CARB 17.1G	
FIBRE 2.8G	
CAL 214	

PECAN & DATE LOAF

PREP TIME: 10 MIN
COOK TIME: 45 MIN

125g wholemeal flour
75g self-raising flour
70g pecans, chopped
6 dates, pitted and finely
  chopped
120ml apple purée
100ml almond milk
  (or regular milk)
6 tbsp honey
1 tsp vanilla extract
20g pecans, whole

This is a bread that is perfect to snack on with a cup of tea in the afternoon. The pecans, dates and apple make a lovely combination. I use readymade apple purée from the health food shop: it's a good ingredient when you want to add sweetness without adding sugar. Dates are real energy-boosters, so a slice of this loaf will set you up nicely before a workout.

Preheat the oven to 150°C/300°F/gas 2. You will need a 900g (2lb) silicone loaf pan.

Sift the flours into a large bowl and mix in the chopped pecans and dates. Mix the apple purée, almond milk, honey and vanilla extract in a medium bowl. Pour the wet ingredients into the dry ingredients and mix well. Pour the batter into the loaf pan. Sprinkle the remaining pecans on top.

Bake for 40 minutes, then increase the heat to 180°C/350°F/gas 4 for a further 5 minutes. This gives the loaf a nice crust.

Remove the loaf from the oven and leave it to cool in the loaf pan for 10 minutes. Carefully remove the Pecan & Date Loaf from the loaf pan and allow it to cool on a wire rack.

PROTEIN 4.1G
FAT (SATURATED) 8.5G (0.7G)
CARB 32.5G
FIBRE 2.4G
CAL 229

ALMOND, PINE NUT & HAZELNUT BREAD

**PREP TIME: 5 MIN
COOK TIME: 3 HR
(INCLUDES SETTING)**

50g pine nuts
50g hazelnuts, roughly
  chopped
250g porridge oats
100g flaked almonds
4 tbsp psyllium seed
  powder
1 tsp fine sea salt (add
  an extra ½ tsp if using
  coarse salt)
3 tbsp coconut oil,
  melted
1 tbsp honey

This is a variation on the Happy, Healthy Bread that appeared in my first book, *Food for the Fast Lane*. Almond, Pine Nut & Hazelnut Bread is packed full of wholegrains and nuts. The psyllium binds the bread, so there's no need for flour. The almonds and pine nuts bring a sweet and buttery flavour to this loaf. Even though I say it takes 3 hours to make, you only spend 10 minutes of that time actually working. So there's nothing to stop you going for a walk or run while you wait for the bread to set.

Blitz the pine nuts in a food processor and tip them into a large bowl. Stir in the rest of the dry ingredients.

Whisk the coconut oil, honey and 350ml of water in a measuring jug. Pour this liquid into the dry ingredients and mix until combined. The dough should be very thick. If it becomes too thick to mix, add a few teaspoons of water until it is manageable. Scrape the dough into a 900g (2lb) silicone loaf pan and leave it to sit at room temperature for at least 2 hours. This allows the psyllium to bind the bread.

Preheat the oven to 180°C/350°F/gas 4. Place the loaf pan on the middle rack of the oven and bake for 20 minutes. Carefully remove the bread from the loaf pan and place the bread upside down directly on the oven rack. Bake for another 40–50 minutes. The bread is cooked once it sounds hollow when tapped.

Place the bread on a wire rack and leave it to cool fully. Store in an airtight container for up to five days. Alternatively, freeze the loaf whole or in slices.

PROTEIN 8.8G

FAT (SATURATED) 28.2G
(10.4G)

CARB 24.1G

FIBRE 13.1G

CAL 417

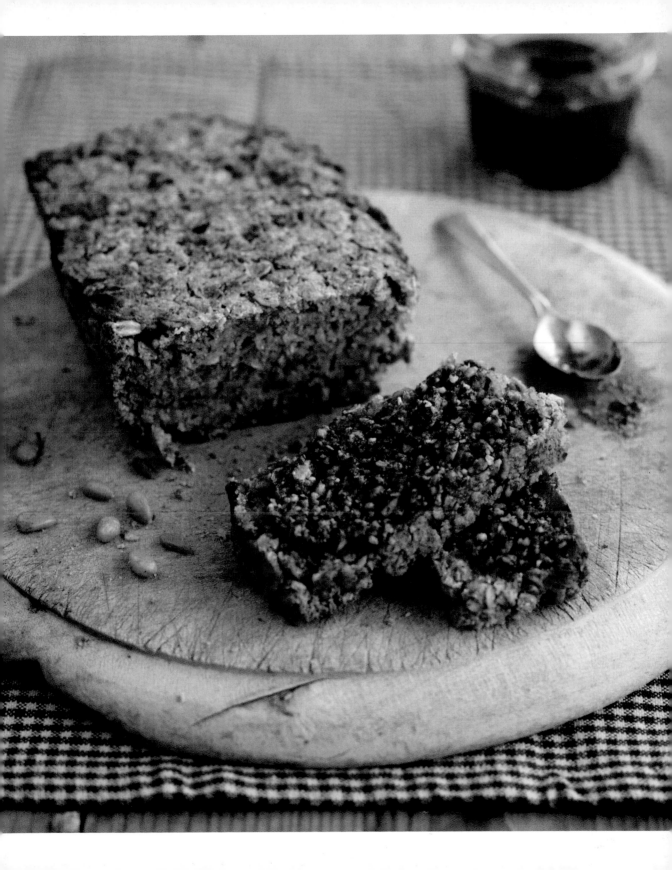

NUTTY BANANA BREAD

**PREP TIME: 5 MIN
COOK TIME: 1 HR
10 MIN**

150g wholemeal flour
90g self-raising flour
2 tsp baking powder
60g chopped hazelnuts
4 ripe bananas, mashed
4 tbsp date syrup
4 eggs
140ml natural yoghurt

A slice of this banana bread is delicious with a cup of coffee. Add a scrape of almond butter or hazelnut butter and you've got a healthy snack to give you a boost after a workout. The date syrup gives a lovely deep flavour but this recipe also works really well with agave syrup, maple syrup or honey. Nutty Banana Bread is great for stocking up your freezer.

Preheat the oven to 160°C/325°F/gas 3. You will need a 900g (2lb) silicone loaf pan.

Sift the flours and baking powder into a medium bowl and add 30g of the hazelnuts. Mix the bananas, date syrup, eggs and natural yoghurt in a large bowl until you have a lumpy batter. Add the dry ingredients to the batter and stir until just combined. Pour the batter into the loaf pan. Sprinkle the remaining hazelnuts on top. Bake for 1 hour or until a skewer inserted comes out clean. Set aside to cool for 10 minutes, then remove from the loaf pan and leave to cool on a wire rack.

PROTEIN 9.3G

FAT (SATURATED) 8.8G (1.6G)

CARB 41G

FIBRE 4.3G

CAL 292

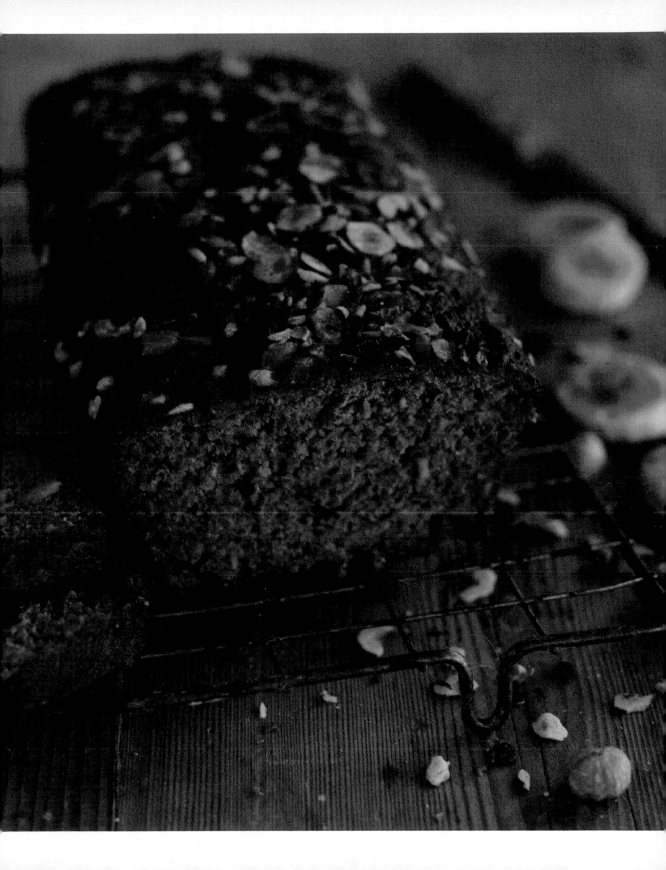

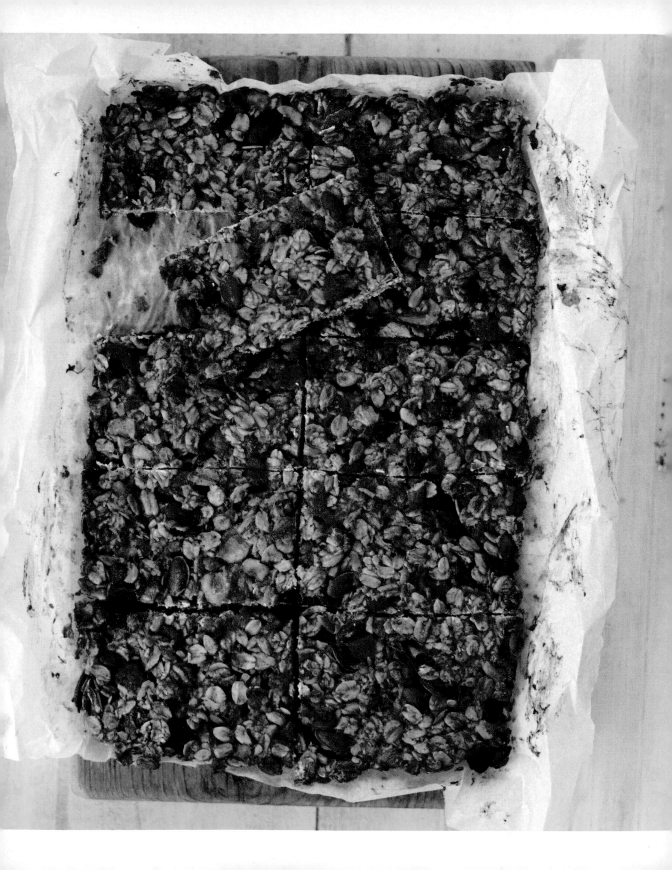

MAKES 12 BARS

BOOSTER BARS

PREP TIME: 5 MIN
COOK TIME: 20 MIN

6 ripe bananas, mashed
120ml agave syrup
2 tbsp coconut oil,
   melted
240g porridge oats
100g dried fruit (dates
   and apricots work well)
60g ground flaxseed
60g hazelnuts, chopped
60g pecans, chopped
60g pumpkin seeds
60g sunflower seeds

Whether you go for a brisk walk, a jog or a full-on session at the gym, there's nothing as tasty as a post-workout treat that you've made for yourself. These bars are particularly good for giving you a boost. The oats are full of fibre-rich complex carbohydrates and the nuts are full of protein. These elements combine to keep you fuller for longer. These bars are far more economical than shop-bought energy bars and they keep for several days in an airtight container in the fridge. If you want to be really organized, you can bake a big batch and then wrap and freeze individual bars. Then just grab a bar from the freezer and bring it in your bag so that you have a healthy treat for later in the day.

Line a 33cm × 23cm metal baking tin with parchment paper so that the paper overlaps the sides. Preheat the oven to 180°C/350°F/gas 4. Use a food processor or whisk to mix the bananas, agave syrup and coconut oil. Combine the remaining ingredients in a large bowl. Add the banana mixture to the dry ingredients and stir well. Scrape the mixture into the prepared baking tin and spread out evenly, pressing down with the back of a spoon.

Bake for 20 minutes, until the top is golden brown and firm. Remove from the oven and leave to cool for about 30 minutes. To remove from the tin, take hold of the parchment paper and simply lift out the slab. Cut the slab into bars and store in the fridge or freezer.

PROTEIN 7.8G

FAT (SATURATED) 20G (5.5G)

CARB 40G

FIBRE 6.8G

CAL 387

COCOA & HAZELNUT BOMBS

PREP TIME: 5 MIN

100g chopped hazelnuts
6 Medjool dates,
   chopped
3 tbsp maple syrup
1 tbsp ground chia
3 tsp good-quality cocoa
   powder
1 tsp vanilla extract

This is my go-to recipe when I want a little snack with a hint of indulgence. I love eating one of these Cocoa & Hazelnut Bombs mid-morning with a cup of coffee or after dinner with a cup of tea. They are also very handy to throw in a gym bag so that you've an energy boost before your workout.

Spread the chopped hazelnuts on a plate and set aside.

Place the dates, maple syrup, ground chia, cocoa powder and vanilla extract in a food processor and blitz until you have a sticky paste. Use your hands to shape the paste into balls roughly the size of golf balls. Then roll each ball in the chopped hazelnuts until coated.

Your Cocoa & Hazelnut Bombs are ready to eat straight away.

PROTEIN 3.2G

FAT (SATURATED) 9.6G (1.3G)

CARB 9.3G

FIBRE 2.3G

CAL 142

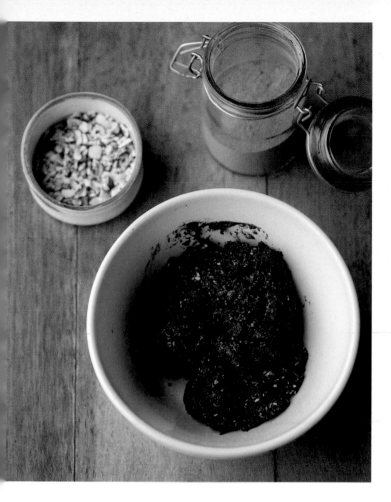

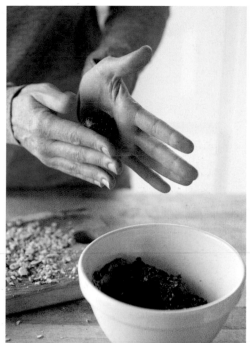

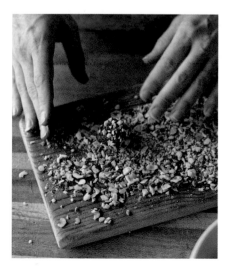

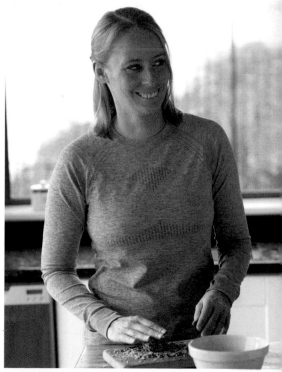

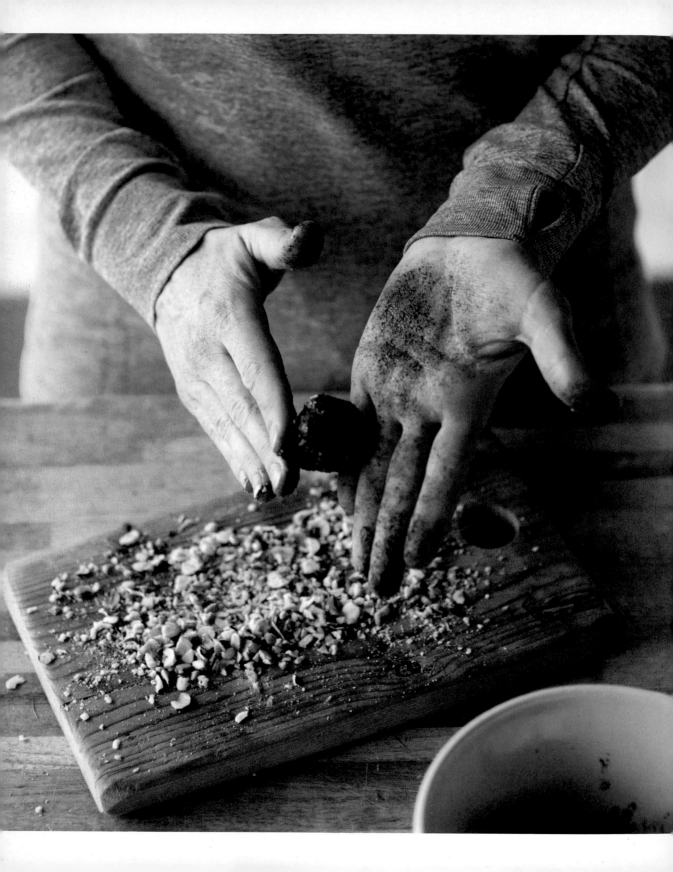

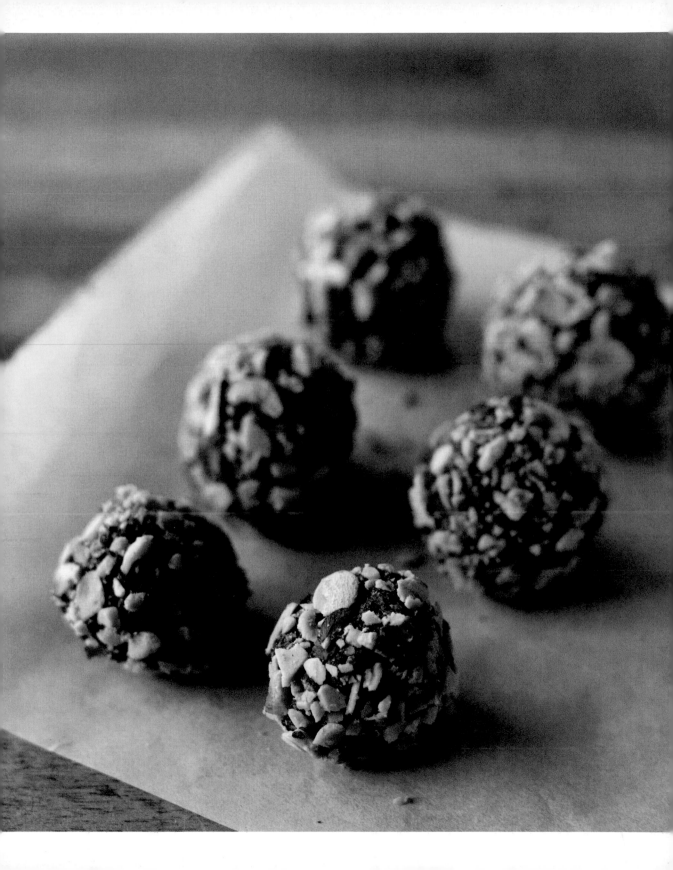

CHOCOLATE & COCONUT ENERGY BARS

PREP TIME: 10 MIN
COOK TIME: 1 HR
** 15 MIN (INCLUDES**
** SETTING)**

170g vanilla protein
  powder
80g jumbo porridge oats
80g seeds (pumpkin and
  sunflower work well)
60g apricots, chopped
60g hazelnuts, chopped
60g pecans, chopped
200ml milk
4 tbsp nut butter (almond
  and peanut work well)
50g dark chocolate,
  chopped
30g desiccated coconut,
  (optional)

I love the combination of chocolate and coconut, so these bars are the perfect treat for me. And they do feel like a treat, even though they've got lots of healthy ingredients in them. It's nice to have a stash of these ready in the freezer. A hot cup of coffee and a cool, chewy, chocolatey coconut bar. What more could you want?

Line a 33cm × 23cm metal baking tin with cling film so that the cling film overlaps the sides.

Mix the protein powder, oats, seeds, apricots and nuts in a large bowl. Add the milk and nut butter. Use your hands to mix these ingredients into a sticky dough. Scrape the mixture into the prepared tin and spread out evenly, pressing down with the back of a spoon. Place the tin in the fridge for at least 1 hour or until the mixture is fully set.

To remove from the tin, take hold of the cling film and lift out the slab. Cut the slab into bars and set aside.

Melt the chocolate in a heatproof bowl over a pan of simmering water. Partially dip each energy bar into the melted chocolate and sprinkle over some desiccated coconut. Leave the bars to rest on a wire rack for a few minutes. Once the chocolate has set, store the bars in an airtight container in the freezer.

PROTEIN 23G	
FAT (SATURATED) 27G (5.4G)	
CARB 13.5G	
FIBRE 7.7G	
CAL 406	

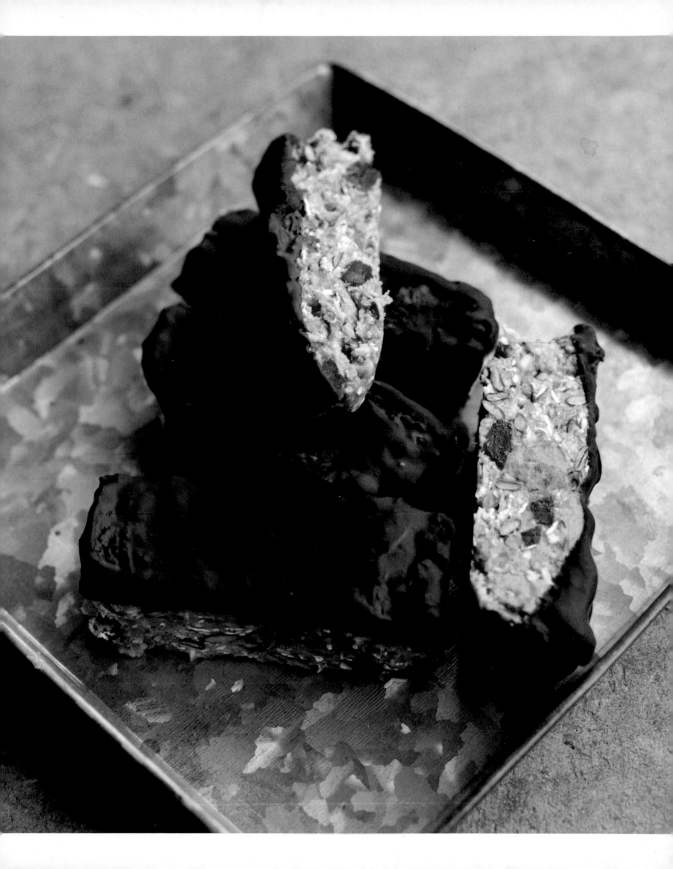

ORANGE & DATE ENERGY BALLS

PREP TIME: 5 MIN

80g desiccated coconut
190g Medjool dates,
   chopped
100g raisins
juice of 1 large orange
120g porridge oats
60g sunflower seeds
2 tbsp good-quality cocoa
   powder

These pre- or post-workout snacks are so tasty that you might need to hide them from friends and family! Whenever I have one of these Orange & Date Energy Balls before a workout, I feel like there's extra pep in my step. They're also delicious mid-afternoon with a hot cup of tea.

Spread the desiccated coconut on a plate and set aside.

If you have time, soak the dates and raisins in the orange juice for 15 minutes before you use them. If not, skip this step.

Place the dates, raisins, orange juice, oats, seeds and cocoa powder in a food processor and blitz until you have a sticky paste. Use your hands to shape the paste into balls roughly the size of golf balls. Then roll each ball in the desiccated coconut until coated.

Your Orange & Date Energy Balls are ready to eat straight away.

PROTEIN 3.5G

FAT (SATURATED) 7.8G (4.3G)

CARB 24G

FIBRE 3.3G

CAL 189

BANANA SQUARES

PREP TIME: 5 MIN
COOK TIME: 45 MIN
(INCLUDES COOLING)

1 ripe banana, chopped
60g porridge oats
25g vanilla protein
  powder (banana flavour
  also works well)
20g dark chocolate,
  chopped
20g desiccated coconut
20g mixed nuts,
  chopped (walnuts and
  pecans work well)
1 egg
1 tbsp honey
1 tsp vanilla extract

These delicious Banana Squares are the perfect pre- or post-workout snack. The dark chocolate and mixed nuts add wonderful texture as well as flavour. Banana Squares can be stored in either the fridge or the freezer. If you like a soft texture, eat them from the fridge. If you want a bit of crunch, eat them from the freezer. Just give them a few minutes to defrost so that you don't chip a tooth!

Line a square 23cm metal baking tin with parchment paper so that the paper overlaps the sides. Preheat the oven to 180°C/350°F/gas 4.

Mix all of the ingredients in a large bowl. Scrape the mixture into the prepared baking tin and spread out evenly, pressing down with the back of a spoon.

Bake for 15 minutes, until the top is golden brown and firm. Remove from the oven and leave to cool for about 30 minutes. To remove from the tin, take hold of the parchment paper and simply lift out the slab. Cut the slab into squares. Store the squares in an airtight container in the fridge or freezer.

PROTEIN 25G	
FAT (SATURATED) 19G (2.3G)	
CARB 9G	
FIBRE 4.3G	
CAL 318	

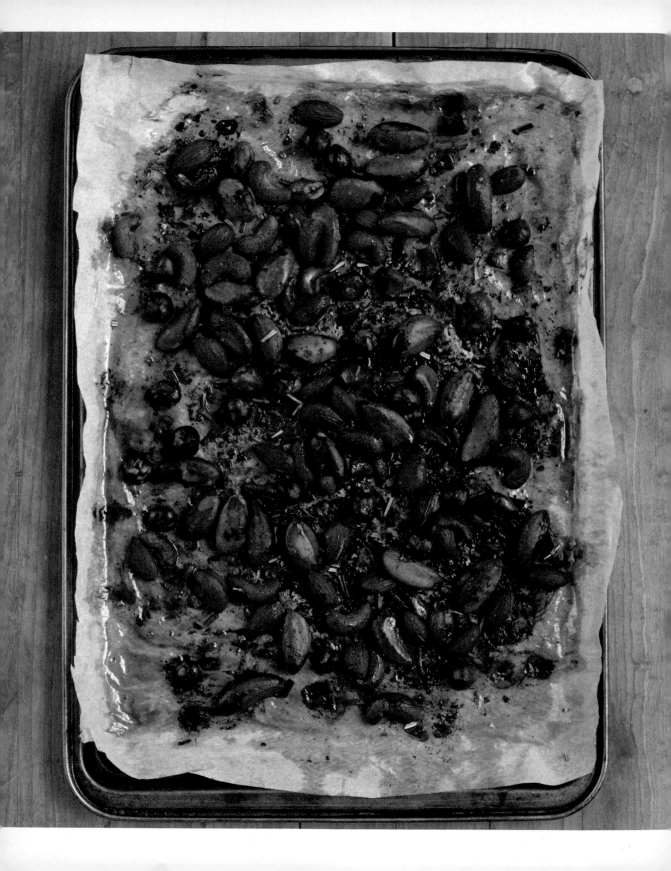

POSH NUTS

PREP TIME: 2 MIN
COOK TIME: 15 MIN

1 tbsp coconut oil
1 tbsp agave syrup
150g mixed nuts
  (walnuts, Brazil,
  hazelnuts and pecans
  work well)
1 tbsp chopped rosemary
  (or 1 tsp dried
  rosemary)
1 tsp chilli flakes
½ tsp sea salt

During my years on the international athletics circuit, I had to do a lot of travelling. I spent so much time in airports and on aeroplanes. I never got to travel first class, of course, and every time I caught a glimpse of the first-class passengers I'd think to myself: *Look at all of those posh people with their posh nuts in first class!* I knew I had to find my own way of eating posh nuts on a plane, so I came up with this recipe. Posh Nuts are now one of my favourite evening treats. They're fiery and delicious and it takes less than 20 minutes to make a batch. You can leave these nuts to cool completely – but if you eat them when they're still warm from the oven, they really hit the spot!

Preheat the oven to 180°C/350°F/gas 4.

Melt the coconut oil in a large pot over a medium heat. Stir in the agave syrup. Take the pan off the heat and toss in the nuts. Stir well to coat the nuts evenly. Sprinkle over the rosemary, chilli and salt and stir well. Spread the nuts on a baking tray. Roast for about 12 minutes, turning once. Leave the nuts to cool on the tray or serve them hot straight away.

PROTEIN 12.9G	
FAT (SATURATED) 58G (16.6G)	
CARB 11.9G	
FIBRE 6.4G	
CAL 639	

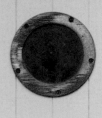

FIT FOODIE
WEEKLY CHALLENGE

A healthy lifestyle is the sum of many parts – it's the combination of a hundred small decisions taken day in, day out, week in and week out. Making sensible choices in the kitchen is only part of being a fit foodie: embracing a healthy day-to-day lifestyle is also vital, and it's incredibly rewarding. I like to set myself small goals that will keep me on track as part of a healthy lifestyle. Here are some of my tips for a healthier week. I hope they inspire you to create your own Fit Foodie weekly challenge.

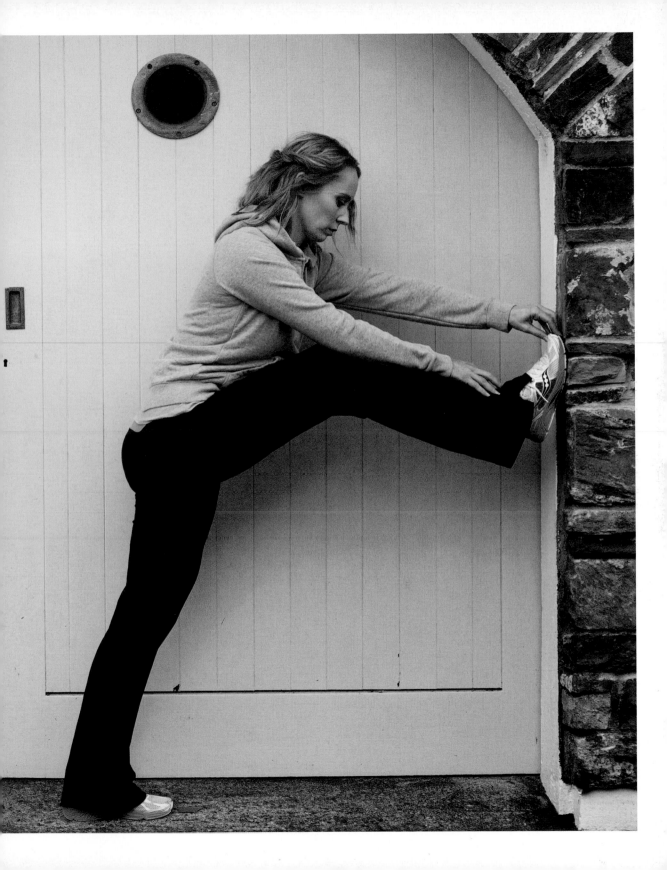

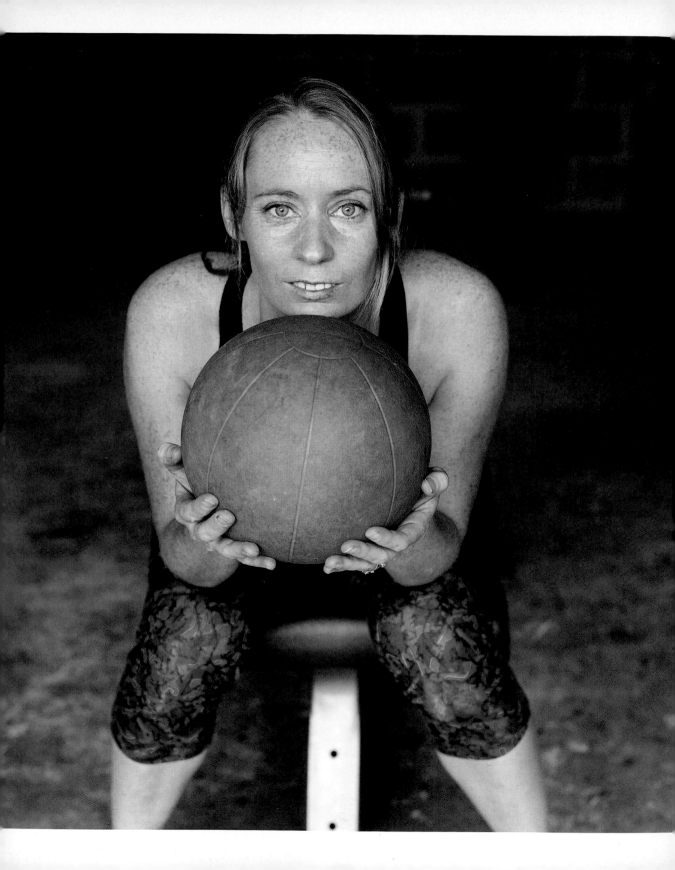

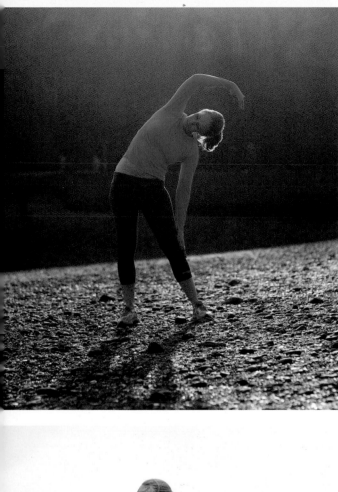

MONDAY: SLEEP WELL

I like to get at least 7 hours' sleep on a Monday night – ideally more. It helps to set me up for the week. Sleep is an essential part of living well and it impacts on everything else we do. I have a sleep-scale as follows: If I get less than 6 hours' sleep, I am dysfunctional. If I get 6–7 hours' sleep, I'm grumpy but acceptable. And anything over 7 hours makes me believe I'm capable of world domination! It's completely unscientific and subjective, but I live by it anyway. I encourage you to prioritize sleep. Get those PJs on and get snoozing so that your mind and body can do some essential recovery.

TUESDAY: LIFT SOMETHING

I believe in the benefits of weightlifting and conditioning. Regardless of what level of fitness you have, a little weightlifting will help. When I'm in a regular routine of weightlifting, I find that it does wonders for my running. I keep a medicine ball (4 kg) in my house and if I can't get to the gym I do a circuit at home with it. Weightlifting is the best route to a toned, strong physique. Try to find a way to work it into your weekly routine.

WEDNESDAY: STRETCH YOURSELF

I spent 20 years running in a straight line and jumping over hurdles, so nowadays I like to find different ways to move. Wednesday night has become Pilates night. Pilates gives me a chance to stretch my body and to challenge myself. Oh, and when I do Pilates, I'm about as graceful as an elephant!

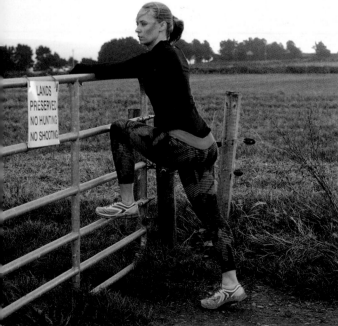

THURSDAY: <u>GET MOVING</u>

You might think that the demands of the working week are not conducive to fitness, but there are always opportunities to move. Try to find ways to build activity into your day. If you normally get a bus to work, why not start walking at least part of the route? If you work in a building with stairs, take the stairs instead of the lift. Honestly, these small changes pay dividends in the long run.

FRIDAY: <u>FIT DATE</u>

When I was a professional athlete, I always seemed to have the time to meet friends for coffee and it never interfered with my workout routine. Ever since my retirement from track and my move into the regular working world, my schedule is not as flexible. So nowadays I organize fit dates! I catch up with a friend while doing a workout. A brisk walk or jog can be a great way to do this.

SATURDAY: <u>BE SOCIABLE</u>

Ask your friends or colleagues if they'll join you for a bit of group fitness. Maybe you can join a fitness class together or set up your own indoor soccer league or tennis tournament. It's good to stay fit in a group because you're accountable to one another and you'll also have a lot of fun.

SUNDAY: <u>RUN</u>

There are few things in life more enjoyable than getting out on a Sunday for a run or a long walk. If you're lucky enough to have extra time on a Sunday, use it to get outdoors so that you can wind down and relax after a busy week.

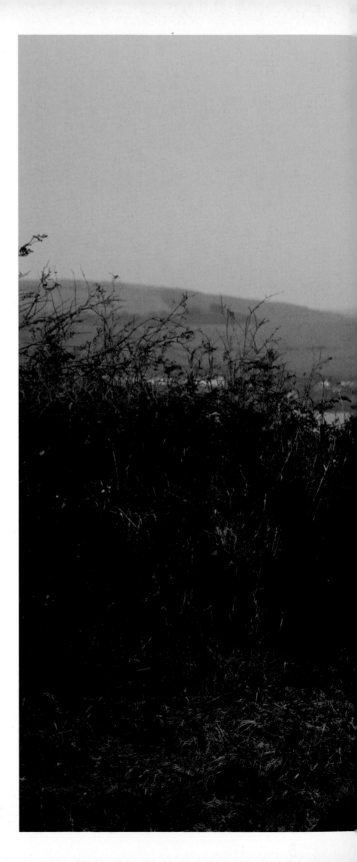

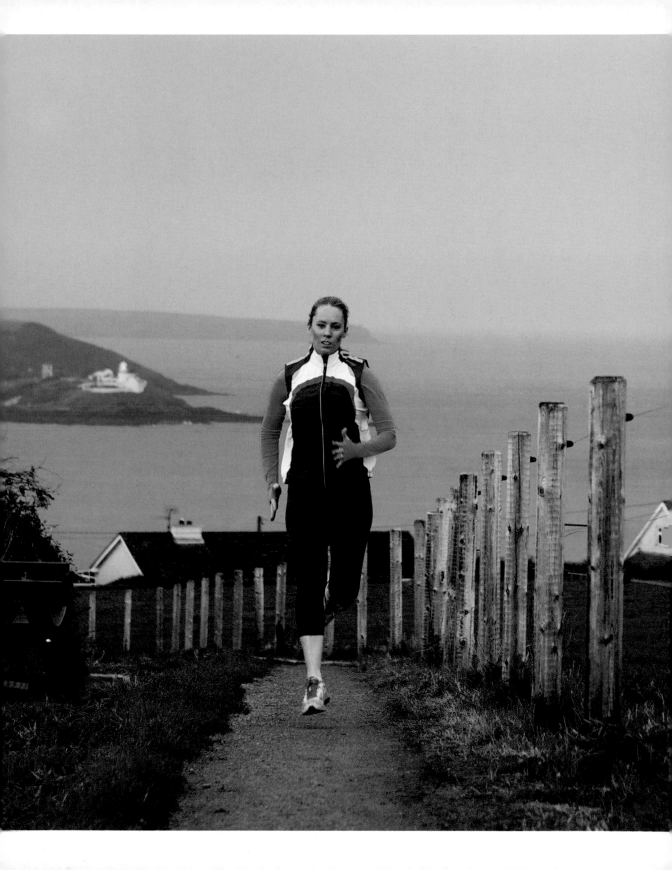

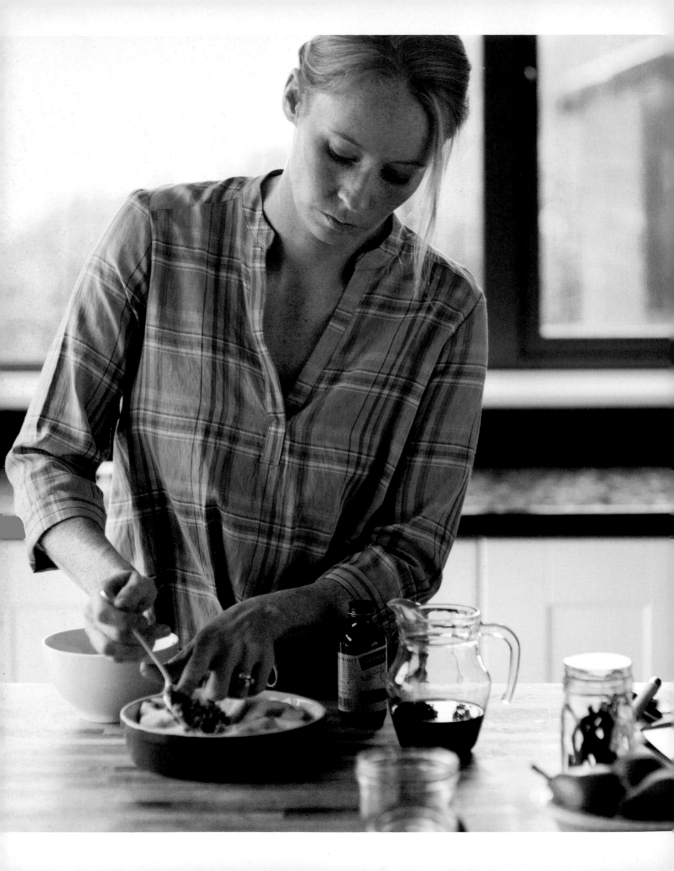

DESSERT

TRISH DESEINE'S CHOCOLATE

FONDANT CAKE

BAKED PEARS WITH

MAPLE & VANILLA

OATY FRUIT CRUMBLE

PINEAPPLE & SWEET

TOASTED HAZELNUTS

COFFEE & HAZELNUT CAKE

TRISH DESEINE'S CHOCOLATE FONDANT CAKE

PREP TIME: 15 MIN
COOK TIME: 25 MIN

200g good-quality dark
   chocolate (65% cocoa is
   ideal), chopped
200g unsalted butter,
   chopped
175g sugar
5 medium eggs
1 level tbsp flour
   (ground almonds also
   work well)
crème fraîche, to serve

I bake rarely – so when I do, I like to make a cake that's guaranteed to be good. This recipe from Trish Deseine (the Irish woman who is one of France's best-known food writers), never fails: it's the only chocolate cake recipe you will ever need. I have happy memories associated with chocolate cake. The biggest title I won in my athletics career was when I was crowned World Champion. The night before I flew to Moscow for the competition, I met my friend and strength coach Martina McCarthy. I had the biggest race of my life coming up and all I could think was: *Wow, I'd really love a slice of chocolate cake right now*. I told Martina, and she advised me to have the slice of cake. She pointed out that one slice of cake was not going to make me any slower. So I had the cake, and I won my title. To this day, whenever I think of my world title I think of chocolate cake as well. It takes massive training and huge effort to win a world title, but a slice of cake every now and then obviously does no harm . . .

Preheat the oven to 180°C/350°F/gas 4. You will need a round 22cm silicone pan. Melt the chocolate and butter in a large bowl over a pan of simmering water. (You can also melt them in the microwave – but do not melt them on direct heat.) Set aside to cool for a few minutes. Add the sugar and stir thoroughly. Add the eggs one at a time, mixing well after each addition, but without beating too much air into the mix. Fold in the flour.

Pour the batter into the silicone pan and bake for around 22 minutes. The cake will be wobbly in the middle. Remove from the oven. Leave the cake to cool completely before turning it out.

Cut the cake into slices and serve.

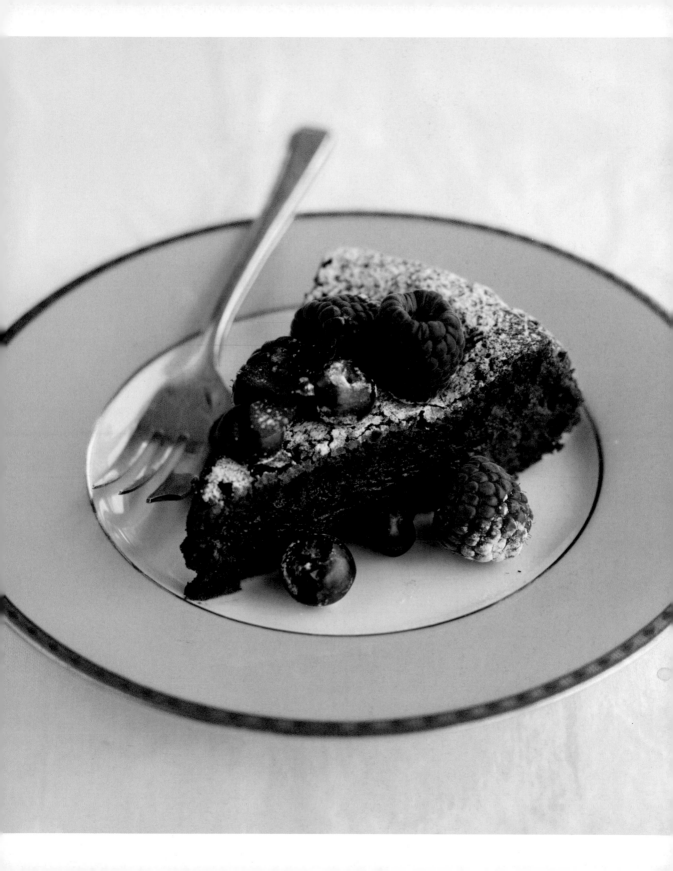

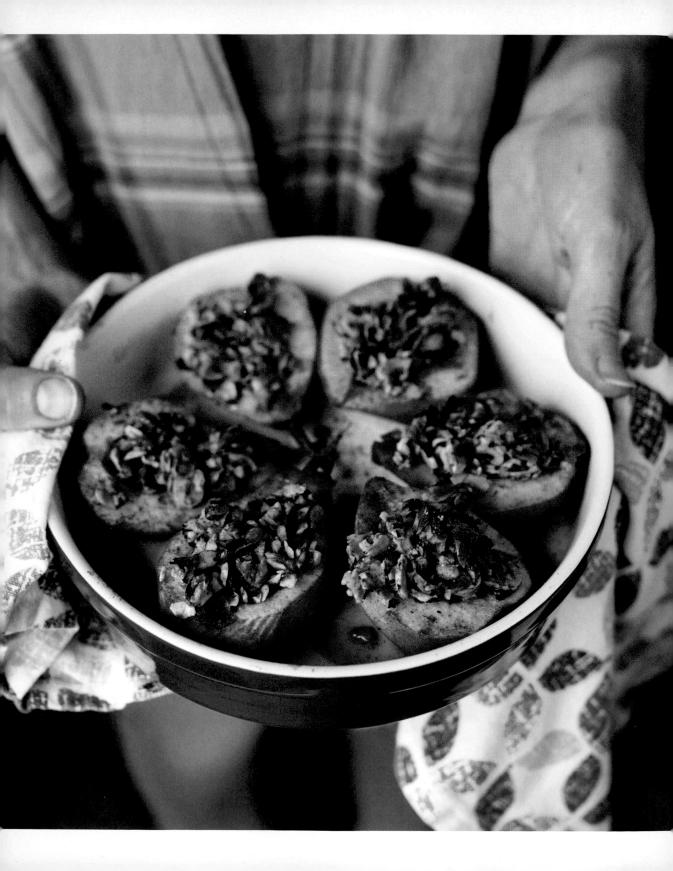

BAKED PEARS WITH MAPLE & VANILLA

PREP TIME: 5 MIN
COOK TIME: 15 MIN

4 tbsp chopped
    hazelnuts
2 tbsp maple syrup
    (honey or agave syrup
    also work well)
1 tsp cinnamon
1 tsp vanilla extract
4 ripe pears, peeled
4 tbsp Greek yoghurt,
    to serve

This recipe is so simple and it makes for a pretty healthy dessert. It's best made with pears that are in season and deliciously ripe – but it's no big deal if you want to use tinned pears. It'll take just 15 minutes for the pears to bake and they will send the most amazing aroma wafting through your kitchen. You need to eat the pears as soon as they come out of the oven – preferably with a dollop of cold Greek yoghurt.

Preheat the oven to 180°C/350°F/gas 4.

Mix the hazelnuts, maple syrup, cinnamon and vanilla in a medium bowl and set aside.

Use a sharp knife to cut the pears in half lengthways. Hollow out the cores using a teaspoon. Slice a little off the rounded side of each pear half so that they sit flat. Arrange the pear halves, core-side up, in an ovenproof dish. Carefully spoon the hazelnut mixture into the hollows of the pear halves. Bake for 15 minutes or until tender. Divide the pear halves between warmed serving plates. Finish with a dollop of Greek yoghurt and serve without delay.

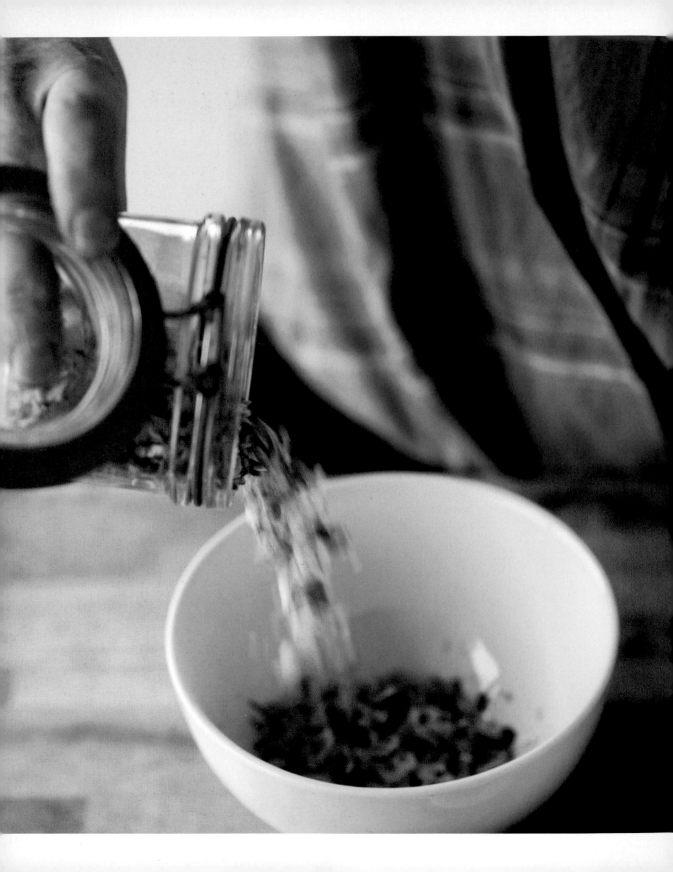

OATY FRUIT CRUMBLE

PREP TIME: 5 MIN
COOK TIME: 50 MIN

2 cooking apples, peeled,
    cored and chopped
100g mixed frozen
    berries (blackberries,
    blueberries,
    blackcurrants and
    raspberries work well)
2 tbsp maple syrup
4 tbsp Greek yoghurt,
    to serve

FOR THE TOPPING
50g jumbo porridge oats
40g butter, diced
50g pecans, roughly
    chopped
25g sunflower seeds
25g pumpkin seeds

This is such an easy dessert: one that you can make even when you don't have anything particularly fancy in the cupboard. Traditional crumble recipes use mostly flour for the topping but I go for oats, nuts and seeds for the extra crunch. I also use frozen berries so that I can make this all year round. Of course, if you can get ripe berries in season, go for it! The crumble is delicious with a dollop of Greek yoghurt on top – for me, it needs nothing else. But if you want extra indulgence, you could top it with ice cream or soft frozen yoghurt.

Preheat the oven to 180°C/350°F/gas 4.

Place the apples and berries in a large pan over a medium heat. Add a few tablespoons of water. Cook for about 5 minutes, until the fruit is soft. Stir in the maple syrup and set aside.

Meanwhile, make the topping. Place the oats and butter in a large bowl. Use your fingertips to rub the butter into the oats, until the mixture looks like breadcrumbs. Mix in the pecans and seeds.

Pour the fruit into a large ovenproof dish. Sprinkle the crumble mixture over the fruit. Bake for about 35 minutes, until the crumble is golden and the fruit syrup begins to ooze up the sides of the dish. Spoon the crumble into warmed serving bowls and top with a dollop of Greek yoghurt.

PINEAPPLE & SWEET TOASTED HAZELNUTS

PREP TIME: 5 MIN

1 pineapple, peeled, cored and cut into chunks

65g toasted hazelnuts, chopped

3 tbsp honey, agave syrup or maple syrup

3 tbsp natural yoghurt

There are only four ingredients in this recipe, but it is so much more than the sum of its parts: it's a true Super Snack! Pineapple contains bromelain, an enzyme that reduces exercise-induced muscle damage and inflammation – so it's a great food to eat post-workout. This snack is quick, healthy, sweet and zingy. And it's ready in 5 minutes flat.

Divide the pineapple chunks between serving plates. Scatter over the hazelnuts and drizzle over the honey. Top each plate with a dollop of yoghurt and serve.

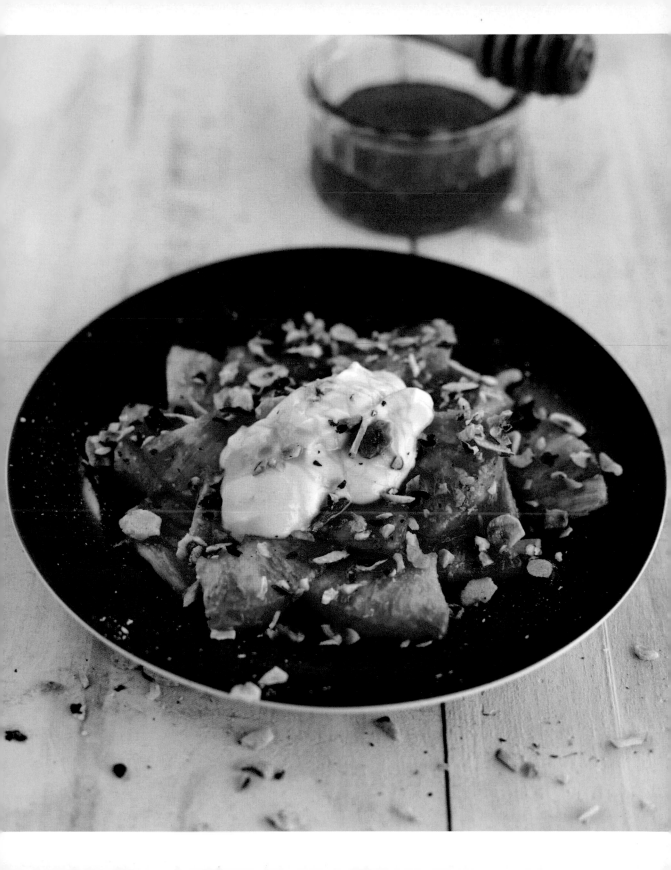

COFFEE & HAZELNUT CAKE

PREP TIME: 5 MIN
COOK TIME: 1 HR
20 MIN (INCLUDES COOLING)

180g butter, diced
180g caster sugar
3 eggs
4 tbsp instant coffee,
  dissolved in 4 tsp
  boiling water
180g self-raising flour
60g chopped hazelnuts

FOR THE ICING
100g icing sugar
70g butter, diced
1 tbsp instant coffee,
  dissolved in 2 tsp
  boiling water
20g chopped hazelnuts

My love of coffee extends to coffee cake – and this recipe is so easy to make. Usually walnuts are used in coffee cake but I like to make it with hazelnuts. This coffee cake is sweet and rich and it's sure to be a crowd-pleaser. It tastes especially good served with a strong espresso on the side.

Preheat the oven to 180°C/350°F/gas 4. You will need a round 20cm silicone pan.

Place the butter and caster sugar in a large bowl and beat until light and fluffy. Beat in the eggs, a little at a time, and then beat in the coffee. Stir in the flour and hazelnuts. (Alternatively, you can place all of these cake ingredients straight into a food processor and blitz until combined.)

Scrape the batter into the silicone pan. Bake for 30 minutes or until a skewer inserted comes out clean. Set aside to cool for 5 minutes, then remove from the pan and leave to cool fully on a wire rack.

Meanwhile, make the icing. Use a food processor or whisk to mix the icing sugar, butter and coffee. Set aside this icing, along with the chopped hazelnuts.

Place the cooled cake on a board. Use a spatula to spread the icing evenly over the cake. Sprinkle over the chopped hazelnuts. Serve with strong espressos.

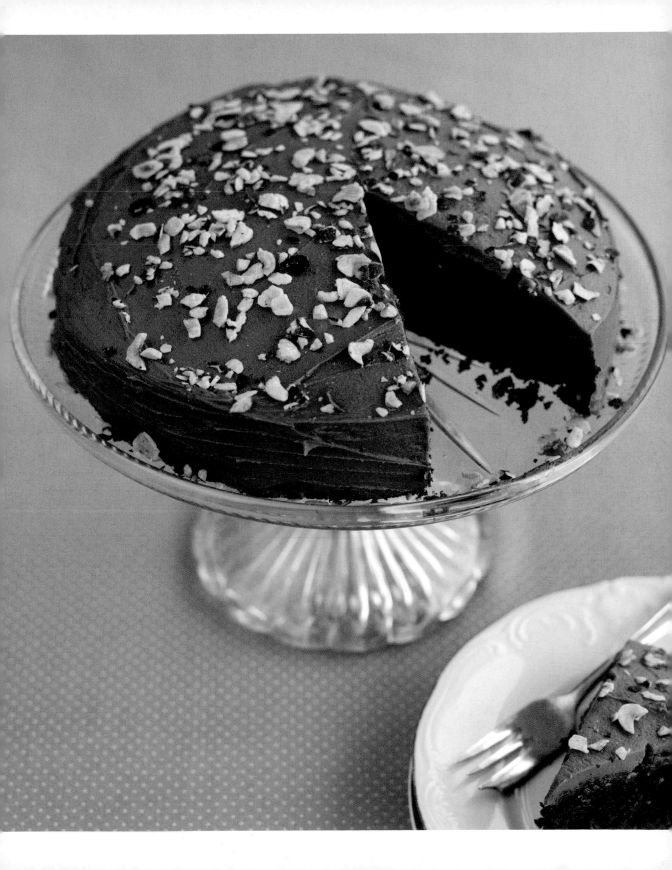

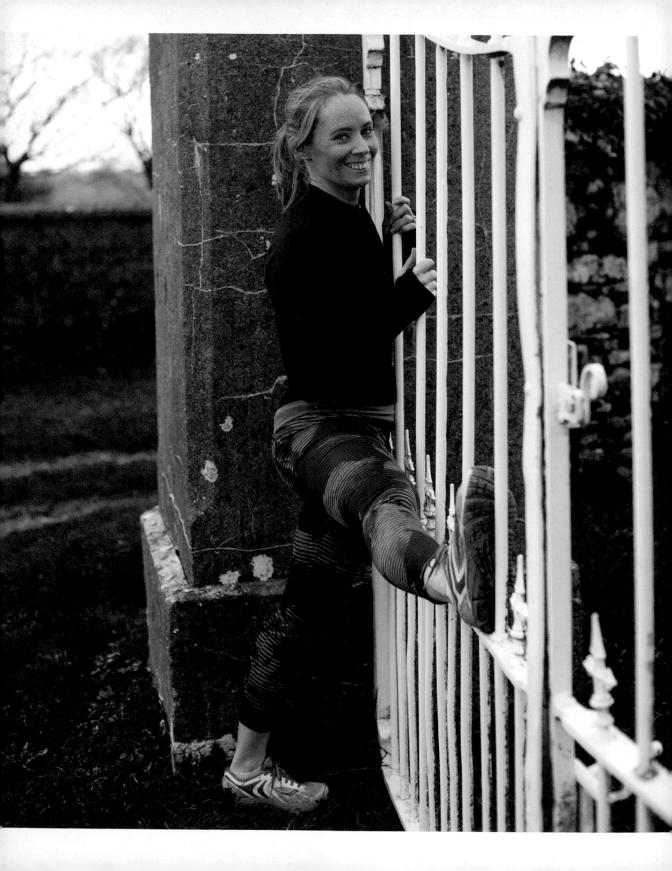

FIT FOODIE FUNDAMENTALS

EAT LIKE AN OLYMPIAN

COFFEE & ATHLETES

KITCHEN EQUIPMENT

FITNESS EQUIPMENT

INGREDIENTS

FINDING NEW WAYS TO KEEP FIT

THE FIT FOODIE PHILOSOPHY

DERV'S PLAYLISTS

EAT LIKE AN OLYMPIAN

SHARON MADIGAN*

Basic healthy eating principles apply to everyone – from a mum doing the school run, to someone running in the park, to an athlete preparing for a big race. Even small changes in what and when you eat can have big effects on performance, health and energy levels. It's about looking at individual requirements. Everybody needs to fulfil basic nutritional requirements first, then vary their diet to meet the demands of work or college (or both) and to allow for fitness training (whether training is daily or a few times a week). Finally, people need to be mindful of any special dietary requirements they have. Here are some guidelines that will ensure you get the best out of your eating and your training:

• COOKING FROM SCRATCH

It would be great if there was a magic health bullet and one food or nutrient that held the answer. Sadly there is no such thing. The simple reality is that cooking from scratch for most of your meals can deliver most of your nutritional requirements. Cooking from scratch allows you to be in the driving seat when it comes to how much salt and sugar you consume, how big or small your portions are, how varied your diet is and the times you eat. These are the cornerstones of any healthy lifestyle. Keep it simple and enjoy cooking and eating well. If you are trying to get into a new routine of healthy eating, a bit of preparation in the kitchen for the busy days can make it easier to stick with. Derval's advice about recipes that freeze well is very useful in this respect.

• COLOUR IS KEY

Including a rainbow of healthy, colourful foods in your diet ensures that it's varied and increases the chance of meeting your antioxidant, vitamin and mineral requirements. You will also be including other essential nutrients such as pre- and probiotics which are crucial for gut health.

*Sharon Madigan graduated from the University of Ulster with an MSc in dietetics and has over twenty years' experience in clinical dietetics. She obtained a PhD in Nutrition Education in 2005. She has worked with athletes across the board – from club and underage to Olympic level. She has also worked up to county and provincial level in many team sports. In 2010 she commenced work with the Irish Institute of Sport where she helps to deliver nutrition services for elite Irish athletes across a range of Olympic and Paralympic sports.

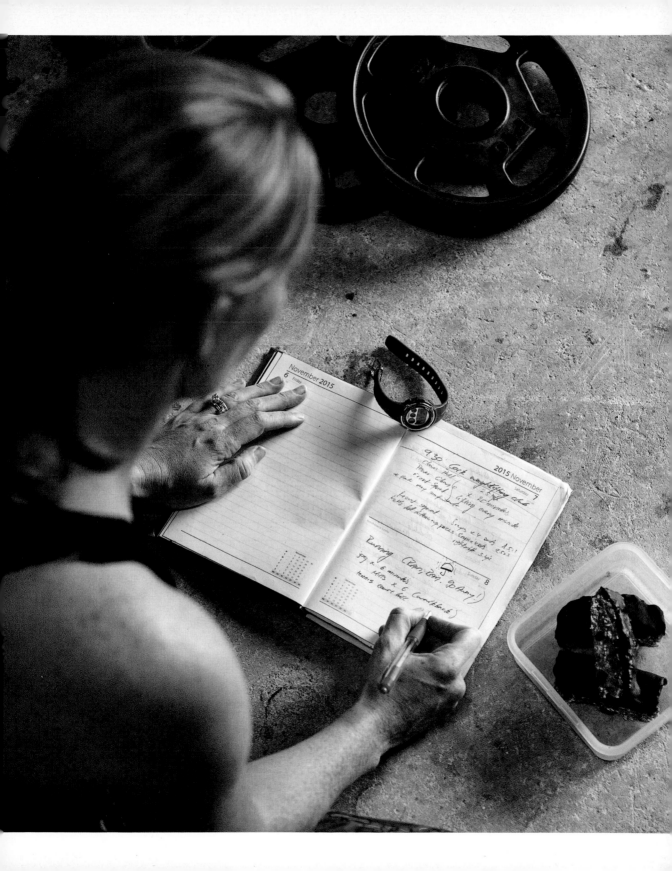

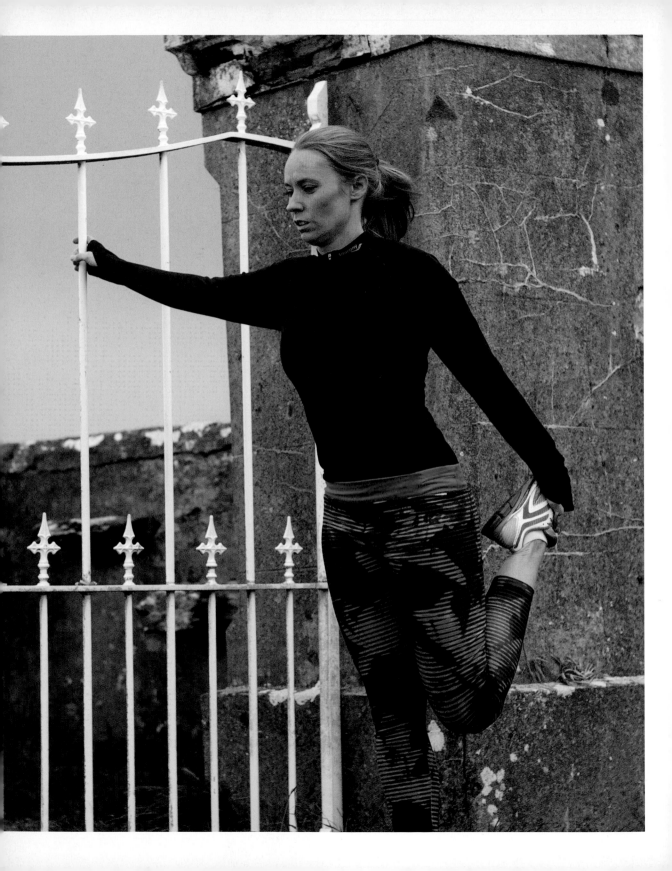

• BE AN ENERGETIC SHOPPER

This is easier said than done – but try never to shop for food when you're hungry or tired. This is where we make poor choices and usually opt for foods that are not as healthy as we would wish.

• NO GUILT

Don't do guilt. If you have a treat, enjoy it and move on. If you are doing the right thing most of the time, then foods that you feel are 'treats' are fine.

• DON'T BE A HERO!

Don't try to make all your changes at once. If you are starting an exercise program and at the same time making drastic changes to your diet, then it will be harder to maintain your new healthy lifestyle. Make changes slowly and you are more likely to be able to stick with them.

• DON'T EAT TOO LITTLE!

If you are exercising or training you need extra fuel. Look at your week: on those days when you are busy and also training, you need to eat enough to do both. Most people eat the same amount each day and then cannot understand why they feel tired or are not getting more from their training. Take a look at some of the meals and snacks in the book that have larger calorie and carbohydrate values per portion. On days where activity is greater, these will offer you an easy option to meet your body's need for more fuel. Making small changes to your food intake to take account of what's going on in your life will make you feel more energized.

FIT FOODIE NUTRITION GRIDS

The nutrition grid for each recipe provides an approximate idea of the protein, fat, carbohydrate, fibre and calorie content per portion as outlined in the recipe. As many of the measures are handy measures rather than exact measures, these figures may vary – for instance, your medium-sized potato could be considered either large or small by somebody else!

These grids can be useful if you are looking to plan meals around training or to give you recovery ideas. If you are going on a long run or cycle, then adequate amounts of carbohydrates are required. For recovery after lengthy workouts, ensure that carbohydrate and protein are part of your meal or snack.

In terms of portion sizes, everyone will be different and the amount you need will be based on what you have done during the day, along with your weight. So a 60kg woman might find that she is satisfied with a quarter of a recipe for, say, stew that provides four servings (the specified portion size fits with her requirements). However, a man of 90kg might need two servings of the recipe in order to be satisfied.

COFFEE & ATHLETES

When I travelled the world as a professional athlete, as soon as I arrived in any hotel I had two questions: *How do I get the Wi-Fi? And where can I get good coffee?* Coffee is almost as important to runners as the shoes they wear!

The life of a professional athlete can be fairly tame and we rely on coffee as an allowable indulgence and a chance to socialize. So at every international competition and training camp, it is easy to find the athletes – find the place that serves the best coffee within walking distance of the hotel and there they'll be. Some of my happiest memories of professional athletics are from cafés all around the world.

Even though I'm no longer a full-time athlete, I still relish a good cup of coffee. Here are my tips for incorporating some 'coffee love' into your day:

- Buy these three essentials: good-quality coffee beans, a coffee-bean grinder and an AeroPress.

- Buy whole beans, since ground coffee goes stale much quicker.

- When you buy coffee beans, check to see what date they were roasted: in general, the fresher the better.

- Buy your coffee beans from a good coffee shop with staff members who are happy to chat with you and answer your questions!

- If you drink a lot of coffee, it might make sense to invest in a fancy coffee machine: get advice from your favourite coffee shop.

- If, like me, you don't want to spend a fortune on a coffee machine, consider an AeroPress. It costs around €30 (£20) and makes one cup of coffee at a time. Over the years, I've asked several baristas what they use to make a delicious cup of coffee at home and the answer is often the same: a simple AeroPress!

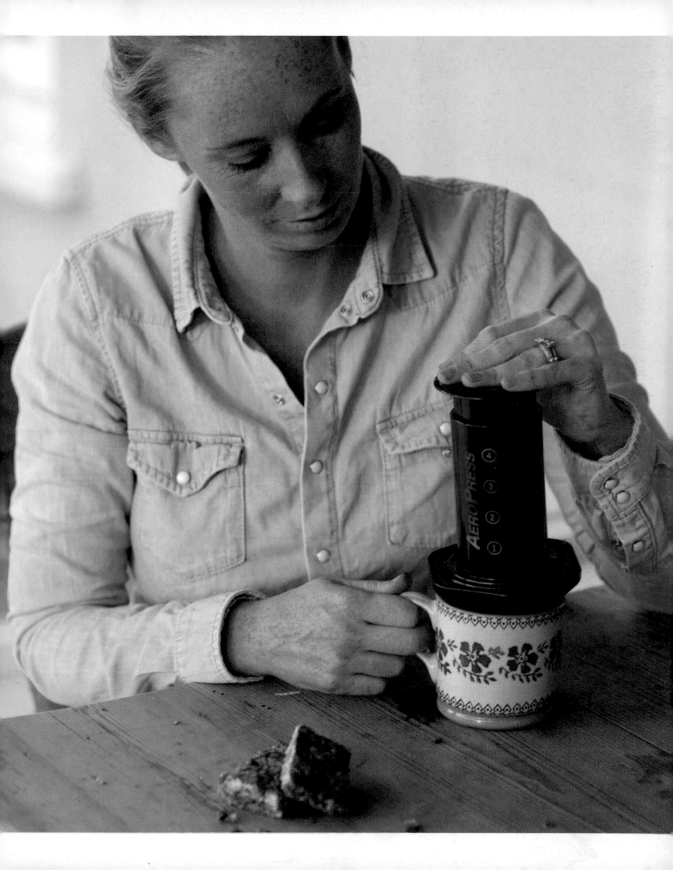

KITCHEN EQUIPMENT

I have moved house a lot over the past ten years, so I have a good idea about the basic equipment that I need in order to cook the things I like to eat. With so much moving about, I've learned to identify kitchen clutter and get rid of it. However, there are a few pieces of equipment that are essential in the Fit Foodie kitchen. Once you have these things, you'll be unstoppable!

KNIVES

I'm a little precious about my knives. A long time ago, I invested in good-quality knives and I believe in treating them well so that I can get the most out of them. I never put good knives in the dishwasher: I hand wash them in hot soapy water before drying them thoroughly.

I've heard this advice many times and I believe it holds true: you really need only three good knives in your kitchen. If you are going to spend some money on knives, invest in these.

CHEF'S KNIFE: 8-INCH

This is the most important knife for food preparation. Before you buy a chef's knife, look at different brands in different shops and ask lots of questions. If you can, ask for a demonstration where you can hold the knife and carefully practise the chopping movement in the shop. I have a Wüsthof chef's knife and look back on it as one of the best investments I ever made. I like a knife with a heavy feel but it's an entirely personal thing. Sharpen your chef's knife as soon as it starts to go blunt.

PARING KNIFE: 4-INCH

A paring knife is used for preparing ingredients that don't need a big chef's knife, e.g. peeling fruits and vegetables. I have never spent a large sum of money on a paring knife. I just find one that's comfortable and replace it once it starts to go blunt.

SERRATED BREAD KNIFE

This is a knife that looks like a saw. Don't bother spending a lot of money on this: but do get one that feels solid. It's the ideal knife for cutting bread, loaves, nut roasts, etc.

FOOD PROCESSOR

The phrase 'food processor' always sounds boring and a bit robotic – but the equipment itself is fantastic and it makes life so much easier in the kitchen. If you can afford to buy a food processor, it's such a good investment. There are endless options out there and not all food processors are created equal. So read the reviews online and ask for recommendations from family and friends.

HANDHELD BLENDER AND ELECTRIC WHISK

If you don't want to spend money on a food processor, a simple handheld blender for soups and a handheld electric whisk will see you through most recipes. My handheld blender was not at all expensive and it is a real workhorse in my kitchen.

OVENPROOF DISHES

Buy good-quality, heavy ovenproof dishes for roasting vegetables, meat and fish. One or two big dishes will cover most needs. Keep an eye out for January sales and other offers and buy a good brand: they will see you through many years of cooking.

BAKING TINS

People bake amazing things at home and there are all sorts of fancy baking tins out there in every conceivable shape and size. I've written my recipes so that the basics will get you through: a few rectangular baking tins and one or two baking sheets are all you really need.

SILICONE PANS

It's such a smart idea to buy a few pieces of good silicone bakeware. Silicone has amazing non-stick properties and is so hardwearing. Invest in a couple of loaf pans so that you can make healthy breads and loaves. And consider buying a square or circular cake pan – just for the treats now and then!

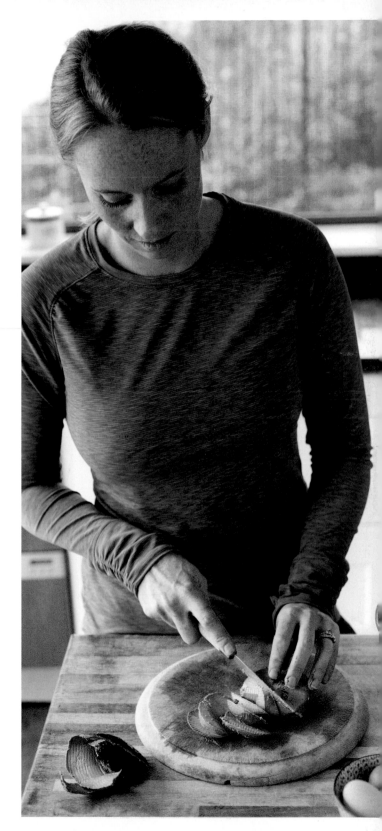

FITNESS EQUIPMENT

I like to be equipped when I'm going to the gym or for a run. During my time as a professional track athlete there were certain items that became must-haves in my gym bag. Pack these into your gym bag and you'll be super-fit in no time!

A GOOD WATCH

The cost of this will depend on what you are training for. I have a basic watch that just times my run. It's a slim, lightweight watch so I don't mind running with it. There are choices out there to meet all needs: get the watch that will help you.

HEADPHONES

I really love music for working out, whether I'm hitting the weights-room or going for a jog. Get headphones that feel comfortable in your ears and won't fall out when you start to move.

GOOD SHOES

I work out in different shoes depending on the activity. I have certain shoes for running, and shoes of a totally different kind for the gym. Good workout shoes will reward you and will help you to avoid injuries. Ask for advice in specialist sports shops.

SUPER SOCKS

There is nothing worse than a bad pair of socks when you are trying to work out! Invest in a few pairs of good-quality, breathable sports socks. They last a long time and the comfort is totally worth it.

BPA-FREE WATER BOTTLE

This is really important for working out. Staying hydrated will benefit you in many ways and drinking your water from a BPA-free water bottle is essential. Plastic bottles have been found to leach toxins into water. You won't have this problem with BPA-free water bottles, which are also kinder to the environment.

THE RIGHT GEAR

It's essential to have the right clothing to suit your activity. A lightweight, waterproof jacket will always come in handy: look for one that allows air to circulate. If you are going to be working up a sweat in the gym, make sure your clothing is breathable and that it fits well.

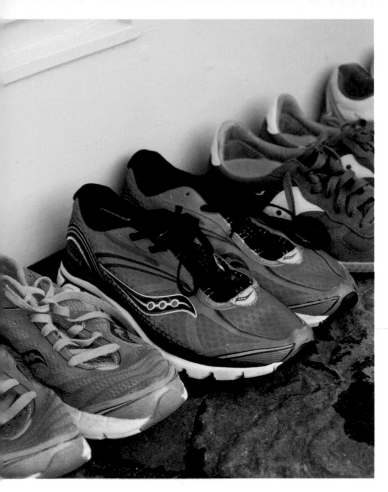

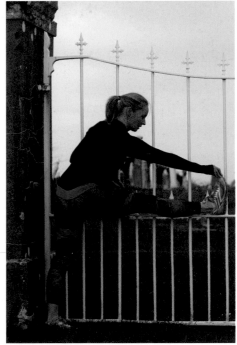

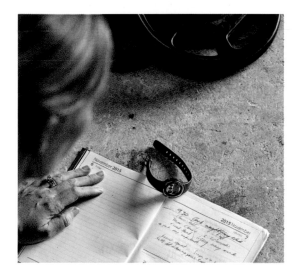

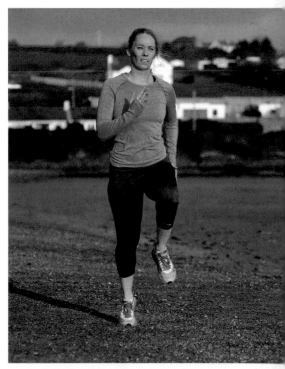

INGREDIENTS

Now that you've read my recipes, I hope that you'll give them a go in your own kitchen! You might have noticed that there are certain ingredients that show up several times in my recipes. Below is some extra information on these Fit Foodie ingredients so that you'll know what to put in your shopping trolley.

BEANS

I think of beans as superhero ingredients: they are nutrient-dense, rich in protein and endlessly adaptable. I have made beans from scratch – soaking and rinsing and all of that – but there's a lot to be said for cutting out all of that work. So canned beans are a must-have in the Fit Foodie larder. While it's true that canned beans are more expensive than dried, the time and effort you save yourself will make the investment worthwhile. These are the beans and pulses that I am never without: chickpeas, kidney beans, mixed beans, green lentils and red lentils. Look for cans without added salt.

CHEESE

Cheese is one of those ingredients that can bring a recipe to life. It really tots up extra points on the taste-scale. Like everything, it should be eaten in moderation. I don't believe in adding lots of cheese to one recipe and then banning it from several menus afterwards. Instead, I add small amounts of cheese to quite a few of my recipes. It's worth buying good-quality cheese: it might seem expensive at first, but a little goes a long way. Most of the time,

I'll have each of the following in my fridge: strong Cheddar, feta, blue cheese and Parmesan.

CHOCOLATE

Good-quality dark chocolate is another larder essential. I like 70% cocoa. Again, a little goes a long way: go for quality over quantity. As well as tasting great, good-quality dark chocolate is full of antioxidants.

EGGS

Eggs are the ultimate healthy fast-food option. I really love them – they are incredibly versatile and are such a valuable addition to meals. I'm lucky that my mother-in-law keeps chickens that live a great life and supply me with fresh eggs. Buy the best eggs that you can afford – free-range and organic, if you can. And remember to bring eggs to room temperature before you cook with them.

FAJITA SPICE MIX

I keep a readymade fajita spice mix in my larder. You can find good-quality brands in your local health food shop or deli. If you

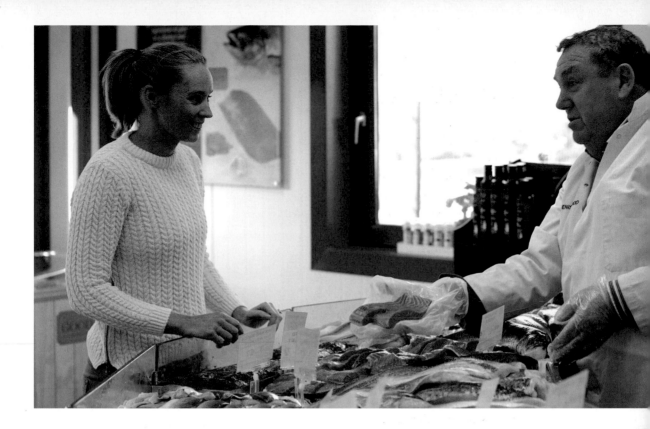

want to make your own fajita spice mix, play around with different combinations of ground spices such as cumin, coriander, chilli powder, paprika and oregano. Find the mix that's right for you, and keep a good stash in your larder.

FISH

I'm really fortunate to live in Cork where some of the most beautiful fish in the world is readily available. My husband, Peter, and his brother, Nicholas, bought a battered old fishing boat and spent months repairing and restoring it to get it back out onto the water. They named the boat *Pelican* and my favourite fish is the fresh fish (usually mackerel) that's caught on that boat.

We can't always expect to have freshly caught fish readily available, so it makes sense to find a good fishmonger. I'm lucky to have a fantastic fish shop a few minutes' drive from my house. If you can regularly visit a good fish shop, it will do wonders for your cooking. Get to know the staff and ask them lots of questions about how to cook fish.

And don't underestimate the value of canned fish! It's an essential ingredient in my larder. I look for brands that use olive oil (rather than brine) on the fish, as it tends to have more health benefits and omega-3 goodness. I keep a good stash of canned tuna, sardines and salmon.

GRAINS

Grains are the bedrock of so many breakfasts, lunches and dinners and they have a long shelf-life. I am never without quinoa, brown and basmati rice. If you're cooking quinoa or rice in advance to be used in a cold salad, remember to cool the grains as quickly as possible and store them in the fridge in an airtight container until you need them. Oats are another staple in my larder. It's worth paying money for good-quality oats: the taste and texture is so much better than cheaper oats.

MEAT

Get to know your local butcher! I have a great butcher who tells me the best way to cook the various cuts I buy and I know that he sources the meat to the highest possible standards.

MILK

As an elite athlete, dairy products were always a part of my diet – and they still are to this day. I always drink full-fat milk because I prefer the taste and I do not believe in completely cutting fat out of my diet. A certain amount of fat is beneficial to our bodies.

NUT BUTTERS

Nut butters will bring life to your larder. A jar of nut butter can seem expensive but it's a wise investment: using just a little nut butter will give a lot of flavour. Read the labels of nut butters before you buy them and aim for as few ingredients as possible. Wyldsson is an online Irish company that makes great products: so many professional rugby players and golfers I know are big fans of Wyldsson and the company makes lovely nut butters (www.wyldsson.com). Meridian is another great producer of nut butters. Meridian products are widely available. I always have almond, cashew and peanut in my larder.

OILS AND FATS FOR COOKING

I use different oils/fats for different purposes in cooking. I invest in three different kinds: olive oil, coconut oil and butter. For olive oil, I buy the best-quality extra virgin olive oil that I can afford. I also love raw coconut oil – and I choose a refined oil with a high smoking-point and no coconut taste (so that it's more versatile for cooking). And when it comes to butter, buy good-quality real butter and use a little at a time.

PESTO

Pestos are easy to make. This is what I do: grab a bunch of basil leaves and blitz it with a handful of shelled pistachios or pine nuts, a little olive oil and some freshly grated Parmesan. That's all there is to it! (You can, of course, make it by hand with a mortar and pestle, but it's a lot slower.) It's also a smart move to keep some good-quality readymade pesto in your fridge. When buying readymade pesto, read the label and ensure that the ingredients list is a short one!

PROTEIN POWDERS

Ideally, if your workout is a strenuous one, you should eat protein within

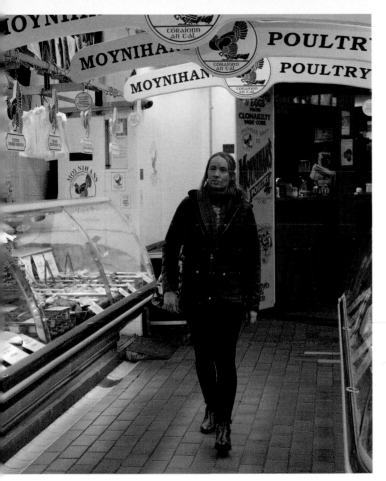
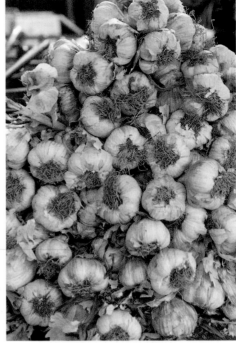
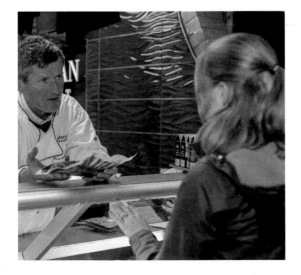
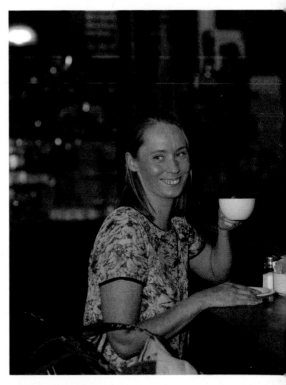

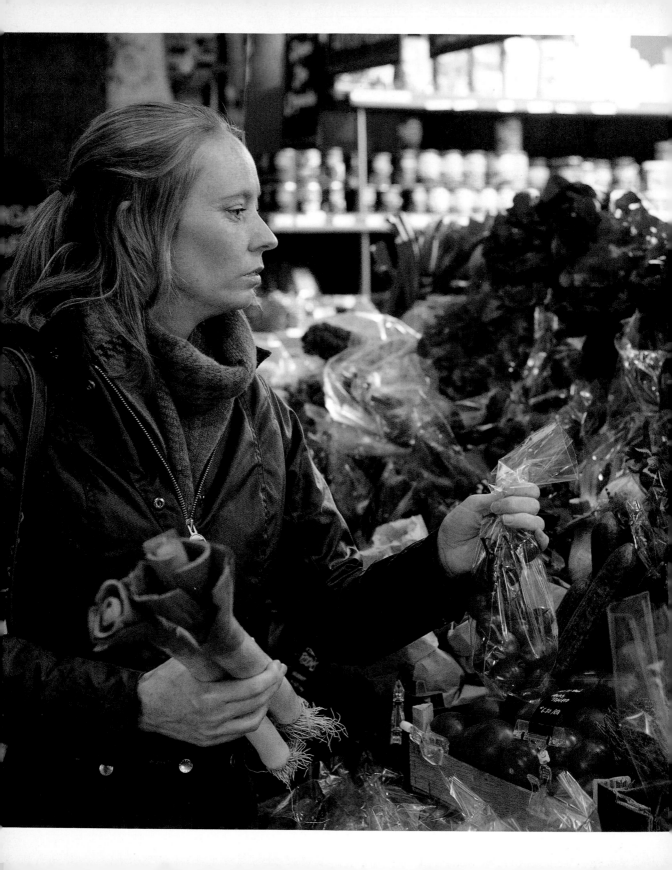

30-40 minutes of finishing. Of course, it's not always possible to get home and cook fresh food within this time. That's why I use protein powder to make healthy bars and treats that I can throw into my gym bag and enjoy as a post-training recovery snack. I use good-quality whey protein, since it's absorbed quickly and helps my body to recover.

SALSA

Homemade tomato salsa is ready in minutes and it can really perk up a meal. I use chopped fresh tomatoes as a base (but a can of chopped tomatoes works well too). Then I stir in some finely chopped onion, garlic, chilli and coriander leaves.

STOCK

I keep Marigold Swiss vegetable bouillon powder in my cupboard and use it all the time in my cooking. Homemade stock really adds to the flavour of recipes too. If you have time, making your own vegetable stock is really very simple and it's a useful base for all kinds of things. Roughly chop two onions, two celery sticks and two carrots and place them in a big pot. Add some herbs such as thyme, parsley or bay leaves. Cover the vegetables with enough water so that you can easily stir them in the pot. Cover the pot and simmer for about an hour. That's all there is to it!

SUGAR ALTERNATIVES – AGAVE SYRUP, MAPLE SYRUP AND HONEY

I use these three sugar alternatives to sweeten my recipes. Agave syrup is sweeter than maple syrup or honey. It's good to remember this when you cook with agave syrup: you need only a small amount.

TOMATOES

Tomatoes are a key ingredient in so many of my recipes. When it comes to growing tomatoes, I've had a mixed experience: I've had beautiful crops and miserable ones! For this reason, I take a fairly relaxed approach to tomatoes. In an ideal world, we would all cook with fresh organic tomatoes. But since this isn't always a possibility, canned tomatoes come to the rescue. Make sure that canned tomatoes come in their own juice, as there can be a lot of hidden sugar otherwise. Passata is another must-have larder item. It's an uncooked tomato purée that has been strained of the seeds and skins, and it adds delicious texture and flavour to so many dishes.

FINDING NEW WAYS
TO KEEP FIT

Fitness is a year-round, lifelong activity. Regardless of what life throws at us, it's important to find new ways to stretch our bodies and keep fit. After surgery on my Achilles tendon, I learned to swim because my body couldn't cope with my usual training routine. When I was in the later stages of pregnancy, I just couldn't run with my bump – so I went on long walks instead.

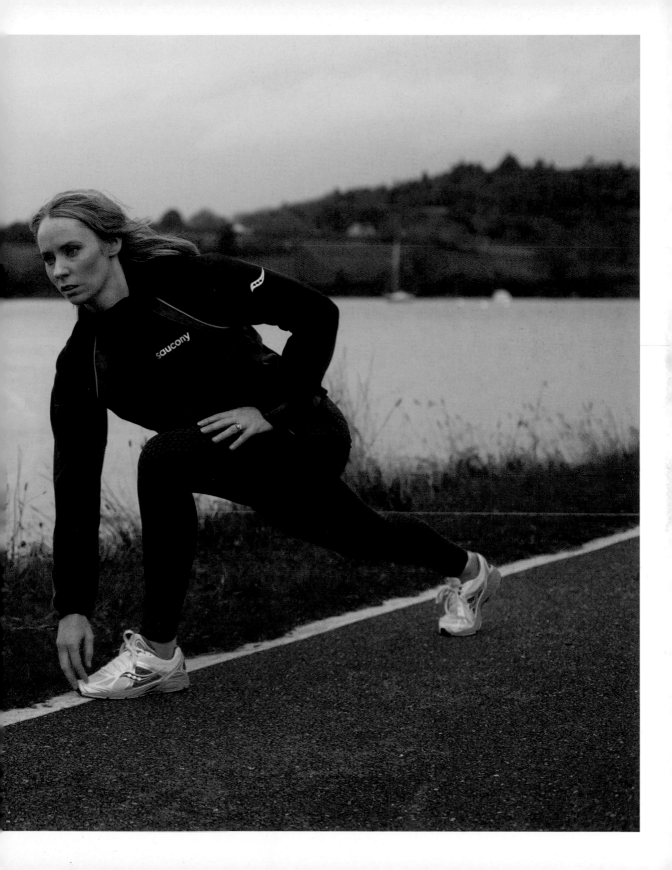

Keeping fit is a mindset. It's about taking it for granted that you're going to do something to move and stretch your body every day. The rest will follow. One autumn, I forgot completely about the clocks going back. By the time I was ready for my run it was pitch black outside. But I was determined to go so, instead of running my usual route, I headed off towards a well-lit housing estate and ran a few loops of that. I'm sure anyone looking out before settling down for the night thought I was bonkers running up and down their streets, but I felt great after the run.

Now and then we'll find that our routine is out of whack and our bodies are different from before. Maybe you're recovering from a sports injury. Maybe you're busy with a young family or working flat out in a new job. If you can't do what you used to do, just lower the hurdle and make a realistic fitness goal.

- If you used to run but it's no longer possible, then walk. Keep moving.

- If you used to walk to work but now you drive, then go for a walk at lunchtime. I bet you have colleagues that would love to walk and chat. Imagine how much more productive you will be after you clear your heads.

- If you used to have a gym membership but now you don't, consider buying some inexpensive home fitness items. A medicine ball is really versatile, a kettle bell is perfect for strength-training and a foam-roller will keep you limber. You don't need a lot of fancy equipment to make a great home gym.

Each of us lives only one life: make sure that it really is the best life it can be.

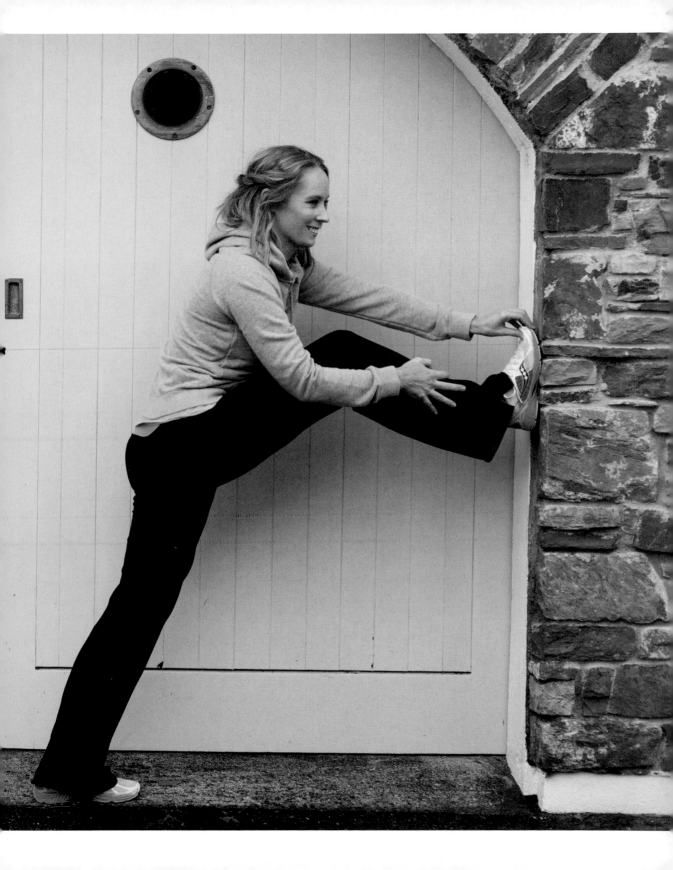

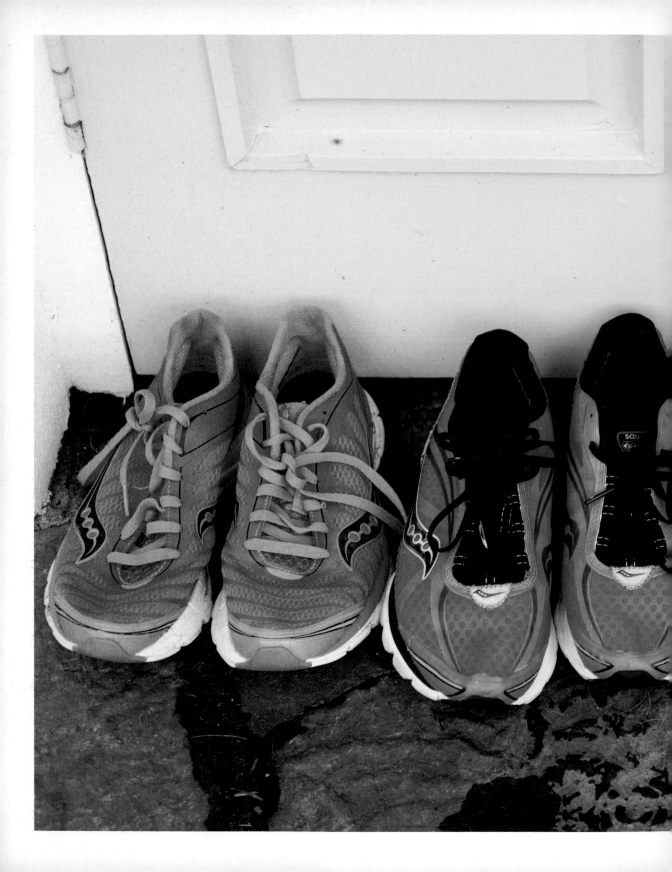

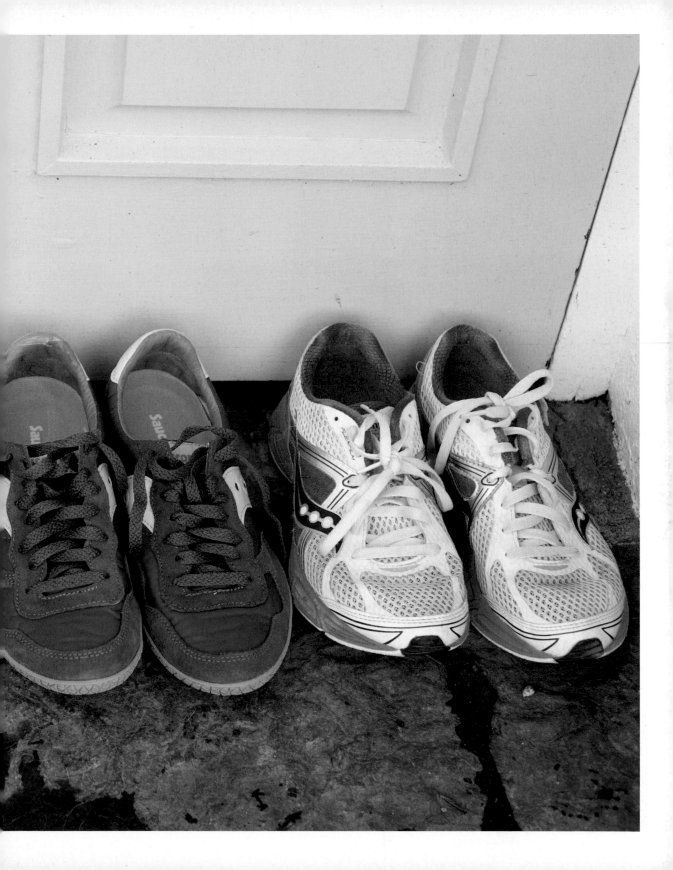

THE FIT FOODIE PHILOSOPHY

Here are some words of wisdom to help you on your way to the Fit Foodie lifestyle.

1 FAIL TO PREPARE, PREPARE TO FAIL
Okay, it's an old one, but it's totally relevant to cooking. Take the time to stock your kitchen properly. Do this and you'll never be caught out with no options for dinner.

2 STAY COOL
Freezer space is valuable: use it wisely. Your freezer can become your go-to place for tasty, healthful, readymade home-cooked meals.

3 SHOP SMART
If you see delicious, healthy food on offer, buy it in bulk: this will do wonders for your health and your finances. Look out for fruits and vegetables in season: get them while they're in abundance.

4 COOK ONCE, EAT TWICE
Dishes such as stews and curries often taste even better on the second day, so it makes sense to cook them in big batches. Fall in love with leftovers!

5 GET YOUR GADGETS
There are certain pieces of kitchen equipment that I'd be lost without (see p. 196). Figure out what you want to cook regularly and then buy a few tools that will help to make your cooking speedy and fun.

6 KEEP A DIARY
Plan your time as best you can – and prioritise the things that matter to you. Jot down in advance the days that you will do a workout or go shopping for ingredients. It's a great way to keep track of yourself.

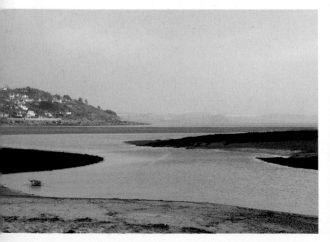
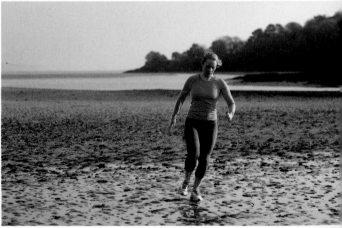

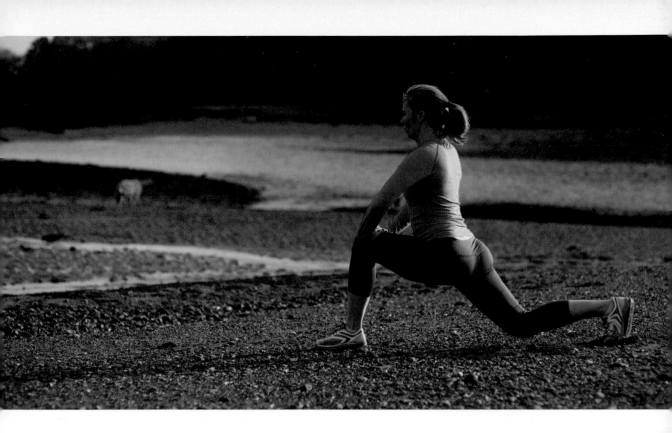

7 DIGITAL DETOX

It's great that we live in the age of the internet but it's important that technology doesn't take over our lives. Put down your phone and go for a walk or a run. You won't regret it.

8 20-MINUTE RULE

No matter how busy you are, you can probably find 20 spare minutes in your day. Use this time to prepare food or to move your body in some way. It will do you the world of good!

9 SLEEP IS SACRED

I love to sleep. Good sleep is such a foundation of good health. Trust me: there is nothing on your phone late at night that is more important than getting your sleep. Put down the phone!

10 CAKE CAN BE THE ANSWER

I don't keep junk food in my house: I would be far too tempted to eat it. I do, however, keep ingredients in my larder that allow me to make a cake at any given time. Sometimes a bit of baking and a slice of homemade cake is just what you need. Life is too short not to make a cake every now and then!

DERV'S PLAYLISTS

I love listening to music and podcasts while I work out and while I cook. Of course, my choices vary depending on which of those activities is on the go!

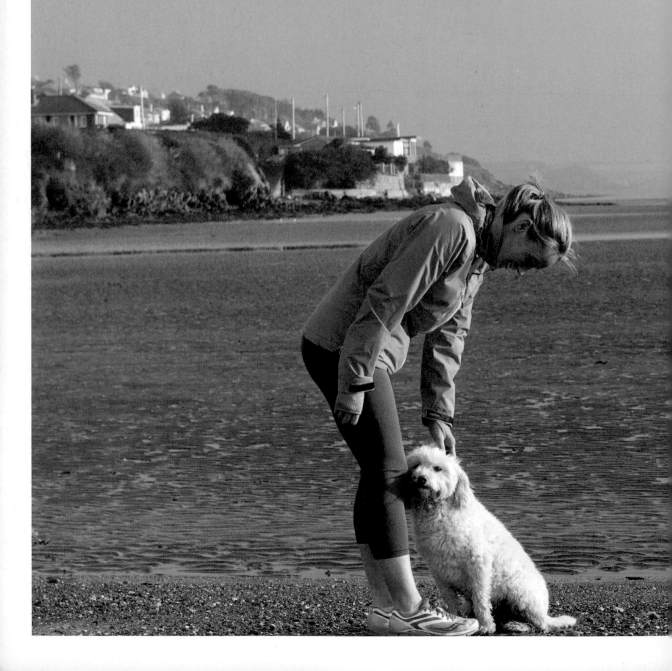

* WORKOUT PLAYLIST *

When I'm working out, I sometimes need extra help so that I can bang out the last few reps in the gym or make the last few metres of a running session. Sometimes you just need a bit of boom in your zoom! These are the tunes that get me going:

- 'Not Giving In' by Rudimental
- 'Money on My Mind' by Sam Smith
- 'Till I Collapse' by Eminem
- 'Do or Die' by Thirty Seconds to Mars
- 'Power' by Kanye West
- 'On to the Next One' by Jay-Z

* COOKING PLAYLIST *

When I'm cooking, I like to have some background noise to go with the clatter of pots and pans! These are among my favourites:

- BBC Radio 4 *Food Programme* food podcast
- *Second Captains* sports podcast
- *Off the Ball* sports podcast
- *TED Talks* podcast
- 'Speeding Cars' by Walking on Cars

INDEX

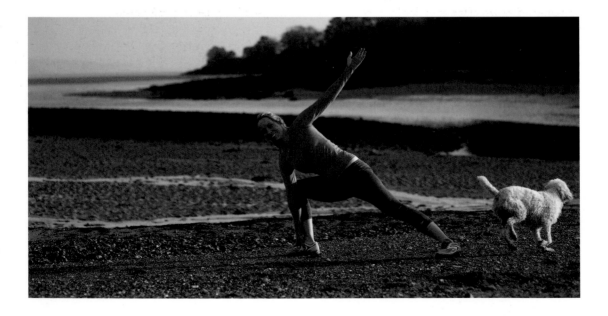

ACKNOWLEDGEMENTS

I would like to say a huge thank you to everybody who has cooked my recipes in the past three years. It has been great to get such positive feedback, whether that's been through social media, bumping into people in the supermarket, on the street or in the gym. When people tell me they've used my recipes, this gives me huge confidence in my style of cooking and recipe writing. It has been a pleasure to go on this culinary adventure: thank you all for making it possible.

I began recipe testing and developing this book over two years ago. During that time I had my daughter, Dafne. The support of my husband, Peter, made it possible for me to get the work done for this book. Thank you for your patience and belief in me. Thank you, Dafne, for being the best girl in the world. I'm a lucky Mama.

My mum and dad, Eva and Terry O'Rourke, had a major role in this book. Their help was incredible. My mother-in-law, Sally O'Leary, deserves to have her name on the cover of this book! She has been fantastic. She has earned her new title 'Challenge Sal'! Thanks to Anthony O'Leary for his creative suggestions!

This book would not exist without the passion, work ethic and great sense of humour of Emma Farrell and Ronan Vaughan of Dog's-ear. They continuously go above and beyond with their work with me. You two are fab and I'm very grateful you are part of the team.

Thanks so much to Penguin Ireland for backing this book. Michael McLoughlin and Patricia Deevy have been great in their encouragement and support. Thanks to Patricia McVeigh, Cliona Lewis, Aimée Johnston, Brian Walker and Carrie Anderson at Penguin Ireland. Thanks to Julia Murday, Sam Fanaken, Sarah Fraser, Keith Taylor and James Blackman for the support and the excitement for this book.

The photos in the book were taken by the very talented and absolutely lovely Jemma Watts. The food shoot was very productive because of your energetic work. Thank you for being fantastic to work with. Cork misses you!

Thanks to Nikki Dupin for all of her hard work on the design of the book – it looks fantastic!

Thanks to fab make-up artist Claire O'Donovan and super hair-stylist Amanda Downey for their work. And thanks to Florence McDonald for all of her help on the food shoot.

I was delighted that Sharon Madigan came on board to contribute to this book. Thank you for being such a fantastic resource and wealth of knowledge. This book is far better for your contribution.

To my great friend Declan Lee, thanks for always listening and coming through with advice and help. A big thanks to Faith O'Grady for getting behind this project. Thank you to Tom Jordan for all the guidance.

Thanks to The English Market in Cork. It was wonderful to be able to show in this book what a special place the market is. Thanks to Denis Good of The Good Fish Company for showing me all your gorgeous fresh fish! Thanks to Tom Durcan Meats for the tour of your shop and the market. Thank you to Tom and Yvonne Durcan: the last-minute borrowing of your kitchen was a massive help!

Thank you to my fantastic friend Karen Shinkins: your recipe testing and feedback is invaluable. Martina McCarthy, your creativity continues to inspire me!

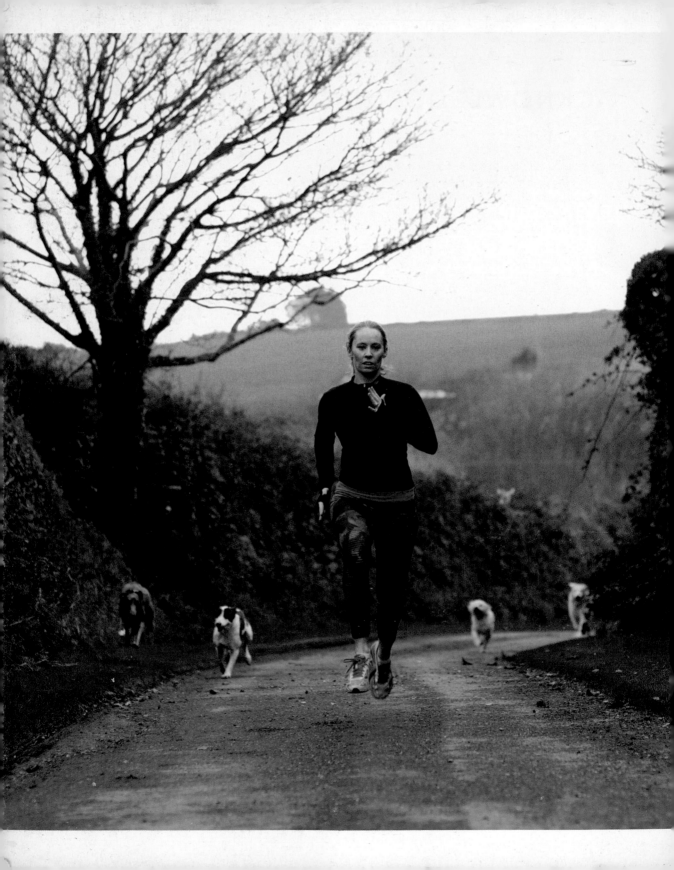